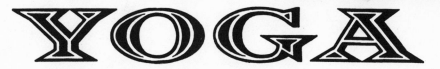

FOR PHYSICAL AND MENTAL FITNESS

Sachindra Kumar Majumdar

Director, Yoga Institute of New York

Stravon Educational Press **New York**

YOGA
FOR PHYSICAL
AND MENTAL FITNESS

PREFACE

In recent years yoga has aroused widespread interest in the West as a method of achieving mental and physical well-being, superior to any known to it. Specialists in many fields—psychologists, psychiatrists, philosophers, doctors, and theologians—have been attracted to its ideas and practices for therapeutic and philosophical reasons. And many of its disciplines, physical and meditative, are being widely practiced by thousands in this country to their physical and mental benefit.

Though yoga has become fairly well known, it is not easy to have access either to teachers trained in the authentic tradition of yoga or to a compact, methodical, and easy-to-follow account of its essential elements. This book aims at meeting the needs of a growing public who desire a concise and reliable introduction to hatha yoga, its beginnings, principles, and practices. It gives the basic exercises of hatha yoga in the context of the broader tradition of the philosophical and meditative yoga.

The exercises are described and illustrated in detail and in all their stages from the first to the final so that they can be easily followed by a student. The various benefits to the exercises are also mentioned.

The book also contains instructive notes on youthfulness, appearance, food, and meditation.

One who follows the book carefully will have a clear grasp of the authentic yoga practices and will be able to follow them easily for his physical and mental benefit.

SACHINDRA KUMAR MAJUMDAR

CONTENTS

INTRODUCTION

Hatha yoga is a system of physical culture and hygiene which originated in the remote past in India as an aid and accessory to the yoga of meditation, the aim of which is to attain transcendental or supersensuous knowledge of self. The goal of the self-discipline of hatha yoga is long life, positive health, and mastery over body and its functions.

Yoga means union and uniting with the higher self of man. It is the realization of our true identity which is above and beyond the little self of everyday life, realization of the self which is transcendental, eternal, and universal and which underlies the surface realities of ordinary existence. Our true and abiding nature is spirit, it is one and infinite, and it is the background or the screen upon which the transient and passing states of body and mind are projected, which gives unity to them and thus creates the notion of a limited and egoistic individuality. Until a man discovers his true identity as spirit he never expresses himself completely or realizes the full meaning of life and human experience.

The desire to transcend the present limits of existence and to know the abiding reality of self is the deepest and secret urge of our life, and this longing becomes manifest when our instinctive needs have to a large extent been satisfied and when we discover the natural limits of their usefulness and validity in the continuous process of our growth toward a deeper and higher understanding and experience. Man's life is basically a life of growth from ignorance to wisdom, from illusion to reality, and from bondage to freedom.

There is only one way of attaining this self-knowledge

or the fundamental truth of existence, namely, meditation or inwardness. Yoga is meditation or focusing the powers and energies of our mind upon the self instead of letting them be scattered and dissipated in different directions, as usually happens. The perfectly inward or concentrated mind is free from distractions; it is still and silent and aware, devoid of dullness, restlessness, or torpor. Such a mind manifests the nature of self in its pristine purity. This is enlightenment, bodhi, satori, nirvana, samadhi, or cosmic consciousness.

There are in each of us—underlying the restless waves of passion and desire, the dull stagnations and gloomy depressions—profound depths of stillness and peace, serenity and wisdom, depths which we can reach through inward meditation. Yoga is the practice and achievement of this awareness.

There are many roads to this destination, the meditative awareness of spirit. All these roads are different forms of yoga. In short, any method which helps to manifest the reality of man from the obscure depths of his personality is yoga.

The yogis, i.e., those who are engaged in the pursuit of self-knowledge through meditation, discovered early that certain physical postures and processes are intimately related to meditative states. They therefore became interested in those postures and processes as aids to inwardness. In the highest meditative state of perfect stillness of mind the various physiological functions are also arrested because life processes are no more than a manifestation of the subconscious psychic will to live and experience. The yogis discovered that all life processes can be brought under conscious control through physical self-discipline and thus made to serve the end of transcendental meditation.

Apart from such considerations the yogis saw that a healthy and firm body and strong nerves were as necessary for the practice of meditation as a clear and rational mind. So they gave much thought to the question of positive health and the factors involved in attaining it. Their aim was not to build bulky muscles and a heavy body but to attain real constitutional health, long life, a strong, slim, and wiry body capable of sustained effort and great endurance, a body resistant to disease and decay.

I
HATHA YOGA

Even a little of this yoga saves one from great fear.

The Gita

HATHA YOGA

Hatha yoga came into existence for the realization of the above objects. Centuries of observation and experiment helped the yogis to develop this into an integral and unique method of self-culture for optimum health and efficiency.

Remarkable health and powers over body and physical functions can be seen among many who practice hatha yoga in India. Many years ago, when I was a young boy living in a small town in northeastern India, there came to my neighborhood a circus party headed by a man named Rama Murti. He was celebrated all over India as a person who had superhuman control over breath and muscles. The circus had animals and acrobats and clowns, as all circuses do, but most special was Rama Murti's demonstration of breath and muscle control.

Rama Murti was rather unimpressive in physical appearance, short and of mediocre build, which his turban did nothing to enhance. But the feat he performed was impressive enough to remain vividly imprinted in memory.

On the evening of the show we sat in a wooden gallery built inside and around a big tent. Rama Murti came fully dressed with an array of medals on his chest. He paused, saluted, and stripped himself bare except for a pair of shorts. He then lay supine on the ground inflating his chest to an astonishing degree, making the chest muscles rigid and holding his breath. A wooden plank nearly two feet wide and ten feet long was placed on his chest. A two-ton elephant then

13

came in quietly from outside the tent, approached him slowly, and placed its feet gingerly one after another on the plank till it balanced itself perfectly. It stayed there for half a minute or so, then stepped back on to the ground again gently.

After that a huge block of granite was placed on his chest and was broken to pieces with a sledge hammer by a muscular man. When all this was over, Rama Murti jumped up and stood and saluted and said that he demonstrated a feat of *pranayama* or yogic breath control.

Muscle control—making limbs rigid like stone, almost stopping heartbeat and remaining buried underground sometimes for days, swallowing deadly poison and ejecting it thereafter by washing the entire alimentary canal by forcing water through it by means of muscle control—can be occasionally seen in India today. However, it is necessary to note that these extreme practices, which are often acts of showmanship, do not have spiritual significance by themselves nor are they favored by the meditative yogis. But they do reveal powers of body one can attain through practice.

The aim of hatha yoga as it is practiced generally in India and elsewhere today is to attain and maintain the body in a state of optimum health and efficiency by attending to the basic factors of health. Hatha yoga discipline builds up a slim and wiry body, well proportioned and capable of sustained effort. It strengthens nerves, improves muscle tone, and vitalizes the body by relieving tensions and releasing trapped energy. Its practice is therapeutic in many ways, as I and many others have observed over a period of years.

The practices by which hatha yoga gains these objectives include postures and breathings with attention to food, fasting, emotions, and cultivation of a philosophical attitude in life. Many who intially approach hatha yoga for purely physical reasons become gradually attracted to the philosophy behind it by the very manner of doing the exercises with attention and awareness. As people become more healthy and relaxed and emotionally stable they become more open to the rational and philosophical background of yoga.

Hatha yoga is an integral or total approach to health. It

aims at the development and self-realization of the whole man and thus involves both body and mind. Proper health depends not only on the growth, strength, and tone of the different muscles of the body, but also on the right functioning of the inner and basic factors of health, namely, the vital organs and the glands.

Techniques of hatha yoga have been elaborated and developed in India through practice over tens of centuries during which the teachers had ample opportunities to observe and study the effects of these techniques on different individuals. Such observations and experiments are still being carried on in India under modern scientific conditions.

All these make hatha yoga a superior and more reliable method of physical culture and hygiene than other modern ones which have not had time to undergo such scrutiny and which, besides, are external and partial in their outlook, neglecting in most cases the basic and essential principles of health.

A fully developed and complete individual is one who has a good mind in a good body. Neither a brilliant mind in a sick body incapable of strong feeling and sensation, nor a superbly developed physique with an empty mind is desirable. Rabindranath Tagore, the famous Indian poet-philosopher and Nobel laureate, said that the complete man should have the vitality of a savage and the mentality of civilized man; that is, he should have a child's capacity for thrill and sensation in its contact with nature while his mind should be governed by civilized values.

Hatha yoga disciplines comprise four broad divisions: 1) posture, 2) breathing, 3) contraction, 4) cleansings. Of these, postures and breathings are well known and widely practised and are adequate enough for a healthy and energetic body.

To maintain health and youthfulness of the body, hatha yoga pays special attention to these basic factors, namely the spine, lungs, heart, and glands.

SPINE

A firm and flexible spine is essential for health and youthfulness. People say a man is as strong as his backbone. The spine stiffens and bends with age, gradually losing its flexibility and springlike curvature. Doctors today recognize the importance of spinal care for health and efficiency. Osteopaths and chiropractors pay a great emphasis on the proper condition of the spine. If the spine loses its natural springlike curvature, if the spinal bones are not properly aligned, and if the spine stiffens from calcium deposits or weakens from muscular failure, our health and efficiency are reduced and we suffer from aches and pains and other unhealthy conditions. Wrong alignment and stiffness of the vertebrae impair the functioning of the nerves which issue out of the vertebral apertures and which control the motor and sensory activities of the different limbs. An increasingly greater number of people in civilized and leisurely societies are suffering from backaches, slipped discs, sacroiliac troubles, and other forms of back conditions, which are often due to bad posture and lack of specialized back exercise.

An erect posture is necessary for proper breathing, healthy body function, concentration, and high emotional level. Weakness of chest and abdominal muscles which come from bad posture hamper normal and restful breathing.

Hatha yoga pays particular attention to spine and the trunk. The spinal exercises make the backbone firm and flexible, strengthen the back muscles, enable the vertebrae to be held in position, and stimulate the sympathetic nerve chains which lie embedded in the muscles alongside the spine.

The various spinal and abdominal movements of hatha yoga energize the basic nerve centers and muscles of the body apart from producing other effects.

Care of the inner organs is more important for health and youthfulness than attention to outward apearances and outer muscles. Of such organs, the lungs are the most important. Breath is life, and breathing is the basic function of the body on which depends the proper functioning of the other organs and the general health of the body.

LUNGS : BREATHING

Lungs need specialized exercise and conditioning, as do the other organs. The civilized man of today, living in comfortable but unhealthy surroundings in many cities, is generally a poor and shallow breather using only a fraction of his lung capacity. Emphysema is fast becoming a common ailment.

As a consequence of faulty breathing, the extreme areas of the lungs remain unexercised and become inelastic and atrophied like muscles which become flabby and wither away from lack of exercise. The air passages which remain stagnant due to poor breathing provide areas where bacteria find easy lodgement and grow quickly. Many colds and respiratory troubles arise from lack of movement and faulty circulation through the lungs.

Shallow and rapid breathing puts a strain on the heart, making it beat oftener than it would. There is a close relationship between the rate of breathing and that of heartbeats. Faulty, restless breathing, even when one is not doing anything, races the heart; it is like racing the car motor by stepping on the gas even when the car is not moving and when the motor should idle leisurely. Deep and rhythmic breathing eases the strain on heart. Many clinics and doctors and psychiatrists employ deep breathing to relieve heart malfunction and to relax tension.

Breathing involves principally two sets of muscles: the intercostal muscles connecting the ribs, and the diaphragm which separates thorax from abdomen. Regular and proper movement of the diaphragm is necessary for the health of the various organs inside the abdominal cavity. Nature intended those organs to be massaged and stimulated by the rhythmic movement of the diaphragm. Without such stimulation the organs do not function well and lead to many troubles. Conditioned movement of the diaphragm and the abdominal muscles helps women to ensure healthy periods and to facilitate natural childbirth.

Oxygen forms by far the major constituent of the body. Poor breathing lowers vitality by depriving the body cells of their oxygen needs. Although it has not been clinically established, some doctors maintain that lack of oxygen in tissues is a factor in causing cancer. These doctors maintain that the body cells which are chronically deprived of oxygen go back to a primitive method of metabolism, and that this causes cancerous growth. There is no doubt that faulty breathing lowers resistance by wearing out the body in many ways.

Age gradually reduces the efficiency of the organs; and breathing power diminishes progressively with growing years. Since breathing is the key function of life, the loss of breathing power inevitably hastens the deterioration of other organs and cells in the body. Breathing exercises retard such processes.

Deep, rhythmic, and controlled breathing has a profound effect on the nervous system and the psyche. Yoga breathing has helped many individuals to get relief from tension as well as symptoms of heart conditions.

Proper breathing improves the form and structure of the body.

Breathing is a bridge between the voluntary and involuntary functions of the body, between conscious mind and subconscious psyche, between body and spirit. Through measured and regulated breathing exercises we can gain a large measure of control over our emotions. Our breathing reflects our emotions and mental states, our elations and depressions, our restlessness and calm. By controlling and regulating our breath, we can do much to relax our nerves, control our emotions, and develop powers of concentration.

Slow and rhythmic breathing acquired through yoga practice slows down the heart and prevents the unnecessary wear and tear of the body and strain on the nervous system. Ordinarily a man breathes 17 or 18 times a minute. One who has practiced yoga breathing faithfully breathes 7 or 8 times a minute. Such slow and deep breathing which is so restful to the body cuts down the aging process of an individual. Most persons age too quickly from wrong and rapid breathing, just as a car motor which races while idling breaks down before its time.

HEART AND GLANDS

Heart disease is the greatest killer today in America. The causes are physical and mental. Diet, no doubt, plays its part but its role has been overstressed. Loss of proper values and the consequent effort to live a life which is against the deeper truth of nature creates tensions, lowers vitality, and damages the heart. When the capacity for love is thwarted by a short-sighted philosophy, a person is denied the kind of self-expression which is necessary for his fulfillment and peace of mind. Such lack of expression or emotional suppression damages the heart.

For good health the yogis emphasized long ago the need for proper emotional expression and for living in harmony with the deep, implicit truth of our nature. There cannot be any true integration and balance between the different elements of our personality without a central purpose of life. This is the function of philosophy—to provide us with a scale of values and a perspective of life. Though ultimately we cannot be healthy without a philosophy, yet physical means are not to be neglected. Yoga breathings and posture remove tension, relax nerves, and improve the functioning of the cardiovascular system.

Glands which control growth and function are deeply influenced by emotions. Most of the illnesses of civilized man are emotionally induced. As heart disease is the greatest killer today, so is arthritis the greatest crippler. Many arthritic conditions, as several doctors recognize today, are due to emotional reasons. Here again proper emotions are so important. The yoga exercises which improve the functioning of the cardiovascular system also improve the glands. Further, there are specific exercises which act upon the glands and restore their prematurely lost efficiency. Yoga food habits are also important in maintaining the health and vigor of the glands.

POSTURES OR ASANAS

The various postures of yoga are mainly spinal, abdominal, and thoracic-diaphragmic movements; they are both dynamic and static. The limb muscles are used to promote effective movements of the spinal and abdominal areas. There are exercises to promote the growth, efficiency, and tone of the limb muscles, but they are supplementary to the spinal, chest, and abdominal exercises.

The postures, especially the ones held steadily without movement, produce circulatory, respiratory, glandular, and nervous changes which increase the vitality and efficiency of the body and create conditions most suitable for concentration, control, and calmness of mind.

The postures and breathings strengthen the roots of the nerves, the brain, the blood vessels, the endocrine glands, and the sympathetic system.

The different movements and postures involve the body in diversified exercises and so tone up all the muscles of the body and keep it well-proportioned, slim and flexible.

For the above reasons and also for others, many whose professions demand a well-kept figure, poise, relaxed nerves, and self assurance, which comes from a healthy and well-balanced body, regularly practice yoga. Many beauty salons are adopting simple and modified versions of some yoga postures for enhancing the face and the figure.

The postures are to be performed slowly, deliberately, without bouncing, and to be held for some time.

The exercises can be done anytime on an empty stomach, but not sooner than three hours or so after a big meal. Morning is the best time, but in cold countries most people find it convenient to do them in the early evening when the body is more limbered up. Regular and punctual practice brings wonderful results to body and mind.

The postures have been carefully illustrated, giving the different stages, from the preliminary to the final, so that they can be easily followed.

NOTE ON THE ORDER
OF EXERCISES

Start with the *Surya Namaskar* and the standing postures.

Next do the breathing exercises in the order given in the book. Assume either the Easy Posture or the Lotus Posture for these exercises except the Abdominal-diaphragmic Breathing, which is preferably done in the supine position.

Then do the following floor exercises in this order: Cobra, Locust, Bow, Back Stretching, Shoulderstand, Plow, Camel, Wheel, Headstand, and Dead pose. Practice time should be approximately 40 minutes.

Add the other exercises as you have time, but keep to the above basic ones. Later on you can practice a few postures for a long period of time one day, and then another group on the following day.

2

EXERCISES
POSTURES
POSES
BREATHING

There is no knowledge higher than self-knowledge. There is no power higher than that of yoga.

The Mahabharata

THE SUN SALUTATION   Surya Namaskar

This exercise combines, in a sequence of 12 brisk movements, several yoga postures and breathings. Many in India practice it early in the morning facing the sun, the visible god of life and energy. It limbers the body, makes the spine strong and flexible, and improves breathing. It also makes for agility and alertness.

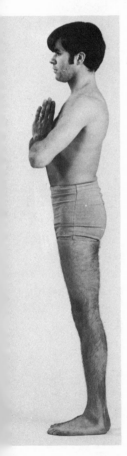 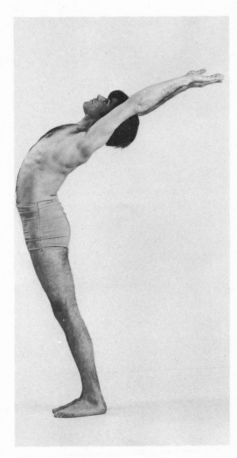 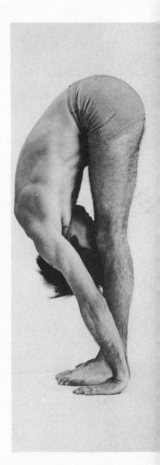

Stand upright, legs together, with hands folded before chest.

Raise both arms, breathe in, and bend backwards from the waist.

Breathe out and bend forward, touching the floor with your hands beside the feet, bringing the head to the knees.

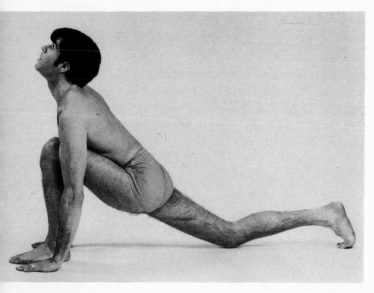

Breathe in and thrust the right leg back, keeping the left foot and left knee between the hands and the arms. Look up and exhale.

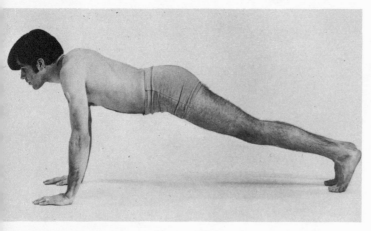

Inhale and thrust the left leg back, putting both feet together, raising the knees off the floor, and resting the body on the hands and feet.

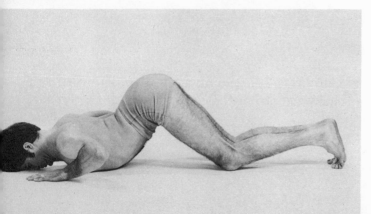

Exhale and lower the body to the floor, touching it with feet, knees, chest, hands, and forehead. Exhale.

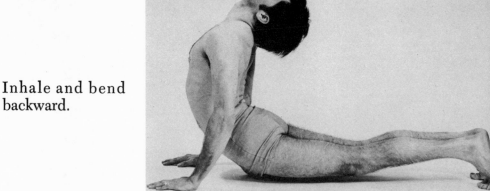

Inhale and bend backward.

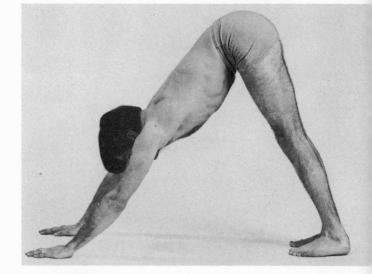

Exhale and raise the body as shown.

Inhale and bring the right foot close to the right hand, with the right knee between the arms, keeping the left foot and left knee on the floor. Look up.

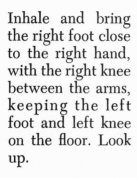

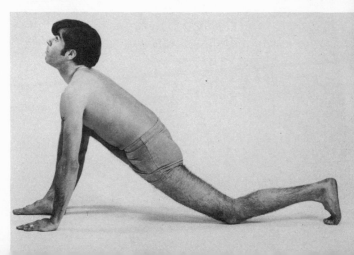

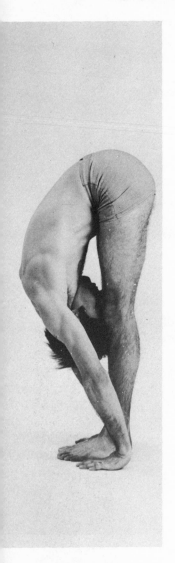

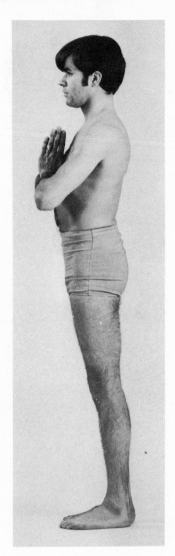

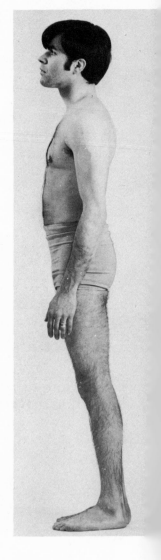

Exhale and bring the left foot alongside the right, straighten the legs, and bring the head to the knees.

Raise arms and inhale as you stand erect.

Drop the arms, exhale, and relax. Repeat 3 to 12 times.

STANDING POSTURES

STAY YOUNG STRETCHINGS   Yuvasana

This is an excellent exercise for limbering up, and for posture and figure.

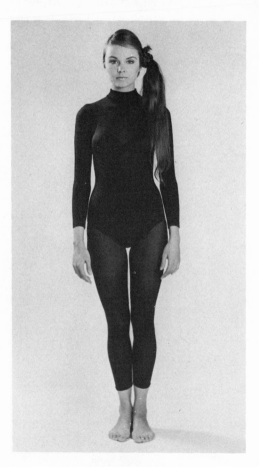

Stand at ease with arms hanging loose on the sides and feet together.

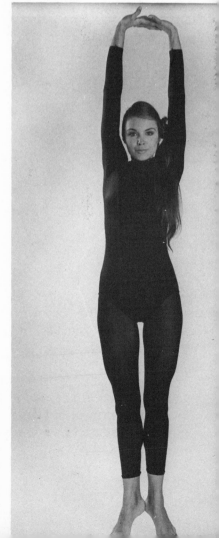

Take a slow, deep breath and as you raise arms over head sidewise, hold your breath and join hands together, interlocking the fingers and raising yourself on your toes. Holding your breath, pull yourself up as much as you can, feeling the pull in your back, shoulders, waist, and legs.

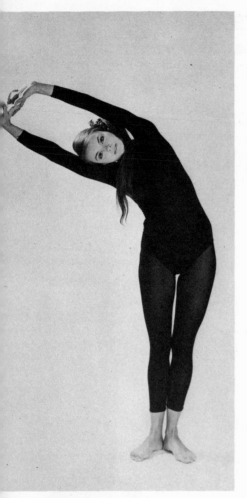

Get down on your heels again and bend to the right side and then to the left, slowly, without moving the hips.

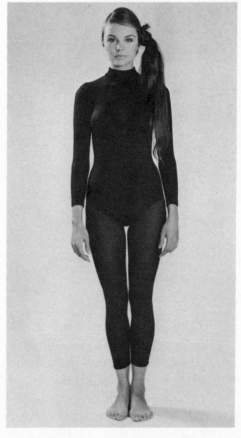

Straighten up, drop the arms, breathe out through the mouth, and relax. Repeat 3 times.

If you cannot hold the breath during the whole exercise, breathe in when you feel pressed for air.

HIP EXERCISE   Nitambasana

This exercise gives proper form and flexibility to the hips.

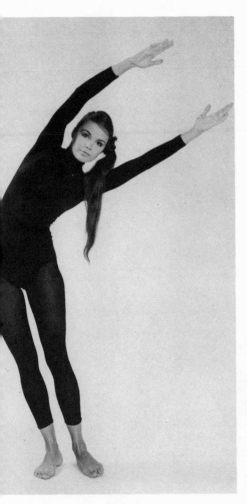

Stand with heels together, arms over head, and palms separate but facing each other. Take a deep breath and bend the body laterally from the hips to the left until it is almost horizontal. Keep the legs straight but push the hips out. Stay in the pose a few seconds. Return to the vertical position as you breathe out.

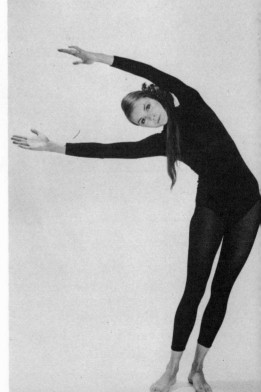

Bend in the same manner to the right. Repeat 3 or 4 times.

TRIANGLE   Trikonasana

This posture exercises the lumbar area of the spine and increases the strength and flexibility of the lower back muscles.

Stand with legs apart and arms extended from the shoulders. Take a deep breath and bend to right, touching the floor near your feet with your right hand. Breathe out as you bend. Stay a few seconds and then resume the vertical position as you breathe in.

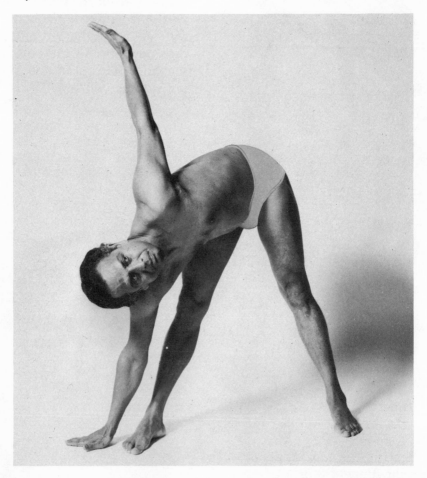

Do the same on the left side. Avoid twisting body as much you can. Repeat 3 times, breathing in through nose and out through mouth.

TRUNK TWIST Vakrasana

This exercises the lower back, abdominal, and hip muscles, and improves posture and figure.

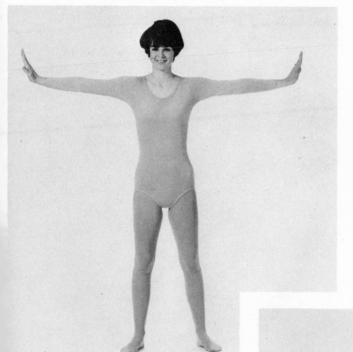

Stand with the legs apart and arms extended from the shoulders. Hold the abdomen flat and take a deep breath.

While holding the breath, twist the trunk right and then left, keeping the arms outstretched. Breathe out through the mouth, and assume the first position. Repeat 2 or 3 times.

KING OF DANCERS' POSE   Natarajasana

This is an exercise for balance, flexibility, and grace.

Stand at ease, hold your right ankle with your right hand, and stretch your left arm up and forward with open hand.

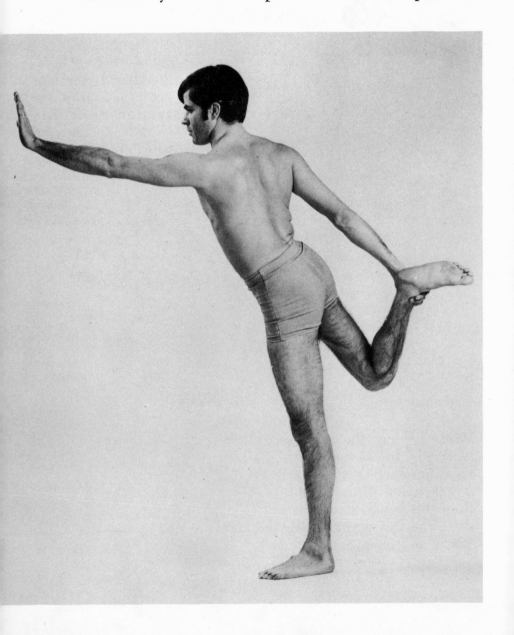

Pull up the knee and the ankle as high as you can, look up, and hold the position for a few seconds. Don't lean forward too much. Do the same with the other hand and leg. Repeat several times.

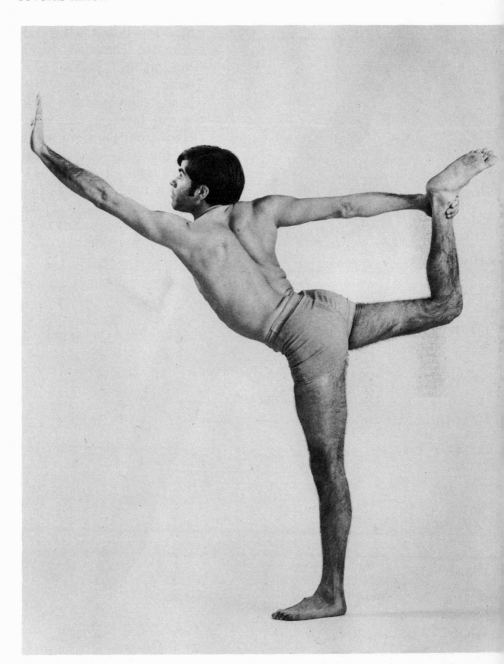

MOON POSTURE   Chandrasana

This is an exercise for grace and flexibility.

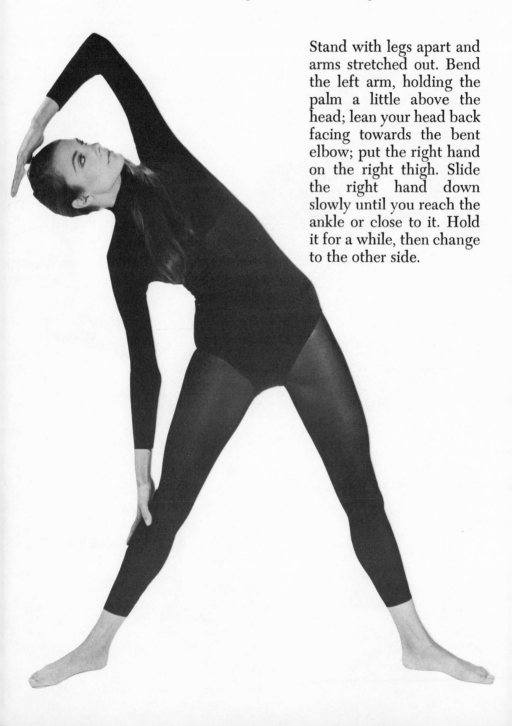

Stand with legs apart and arms stretched out. Bend the left arm, holding the palm a little above the head; lean your head back facing towards the bent elbow; put the right hand on the right thigh. Slide the right hand down slowly until you reach the ankle or close to it. Hold it for a while, then change to the other side.

ONE LEG STAND　　Ekapadasana

This strengthens leg muscles, especially the thigh muscles, and improves balance.

Stand with one leg forward and bent at the knee, keeping the heels on the floor. Stretch both arms forward, parallel to each other with palms facing.

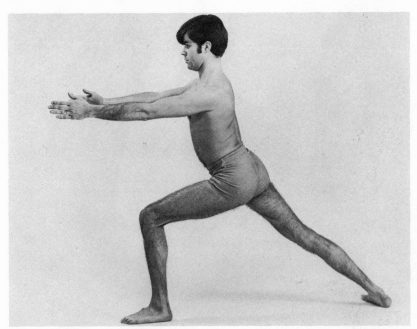

Slowly raise one leg behind and bend forward until you make yourself like the letter T. Hold it for a while. Change to the other leg. Hold the back straight, don't stoop. Repeat several times.

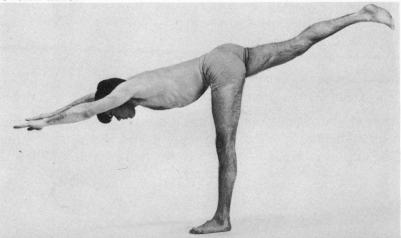

TREE   Vrikshasana

Apart from the benefits of grace, balance, and flexibility, this exercise is especially good for hips.

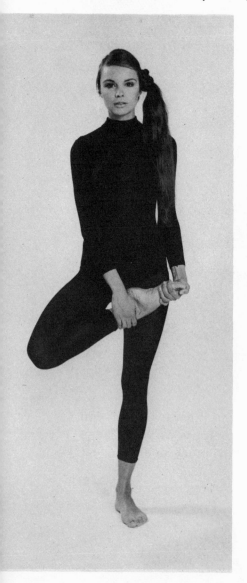

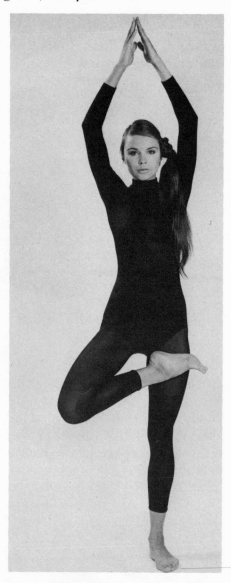

Stand upright, hold one foot with both hands, and place it against the opposite thigh.

Raise both hands, join the palms together, and bend the other knee to make yourself like a chair.

Bring the palms in front of the chest, holding the back straight. Hold a few seconds. Change to the other side. Repeat several times.

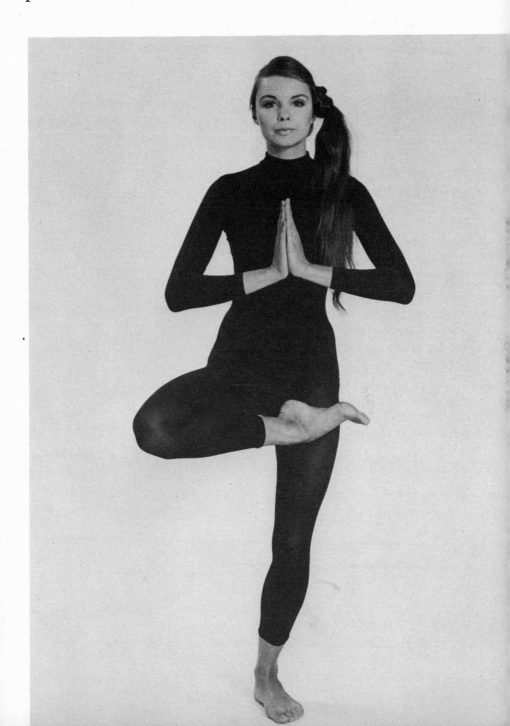

HEAD KNEE BEND   Padahastasana

This important spinal exercise maintains the flexibility of the spine, improving circulation in the back. It also stretches the hamstring muscles.

Stand upright, raise both arms forward and straight up, and bend backward from the waist. Then, bend down forward, breathing out through the mouth. Touch the floor first with both hands, then hold the ankles and bring the head to the knees. While bringing the head to the knees bring the elbows on both sides of the knees as shown. Pull from the hips as you bend forward and keep the legs straight. Stay in the pose for a few seconds and resume the first position. Take a breath as you relax. Repeat twice.

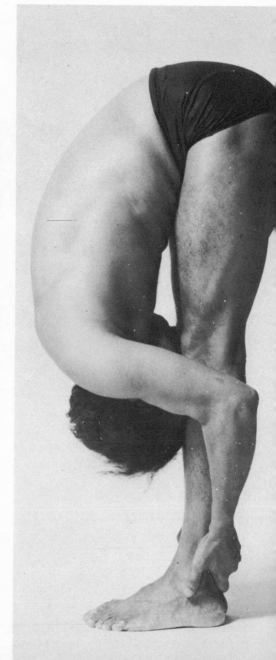

CHEST AND SHOULDER EXERCISE
Vaksha-skandhasana

This posture relieves tension in the neck and shoulders, and tones up the breast muscles.

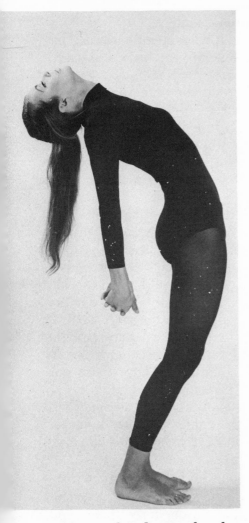 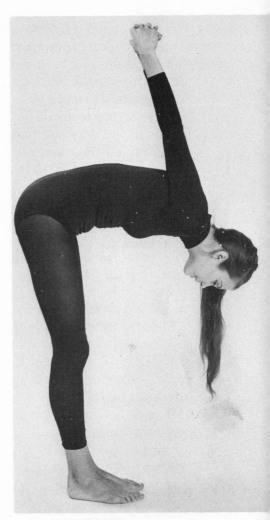

Hold your hands together behind your back and interlock your fingers. Keep the arms straight and bend backward from the waist while keeping the arms stretched out and squeezing the shoulders. Hold it for a few seconds.

Bend forward and down, raising the arms over head. Bring the head as close to the knees as possible. Breathe in while bending backward and breathe out while bending forward. Repeat several times.

SITTING AND
BREATHING EXERCISES

The importance of yoga breathing exercises and the benefits to be derived from them cannot be overemphasized. They should be done with attention, keeping the body still except for the muscles directly involved.

Breathing exercises should be done on an empty stomach.

It is advisable to do a few stretching and limbering exercises in the standing position before starting the breathing exercises. This is especially important in cold weather.

Have plenty of fresh air in the room when you exercise but avoid drafts. It is excellent to do them in the open in warm weather.

Most breathing exercises are done in a sitting position, in the Easy Posture or the Lotus Posture. The spine should be held erect, in line with the neck and the head. The chest should be thrust forward a bit as if the weight of the body is supported by the ribs. The clothing should be loose and should not press against the body; better without it altogether.

Those who are unable to sit properly in the yoga postures may sit in a chair, but should always hold the back straight.

The Easy Posture and Lotus Posture are recommended by yogis for concentration and meditation because these postures can be held with ease for prolonged meditation.

It may not be easy for some Westerners to assume these positions in the beginning. With regular practice, however, it will become less difficult for most to assume first the Easy Posture and then the Lotus Posture.

If you find it difficult to assume the Easy Posture, sit as a tailor does, with legs crossed and back straight. The knees will gradually become limber, but do not force them. And, learn the habit of sitting in that position whenever you read or eat.

To keep the back straight and the knees down, some may find it helpful to sit on a hassock or a pillow, keeping the knees outspread and off the pillow. Only the buttocks should rest on the pillow.

EASY POSTURE   Sukhasana

This posture, held for a long period of time, aids concentration and has beneficial psychological and physical effects, promoting a high level of thought and well-being.

Sit on the floor with both legs stretched. Bend the right leg and bring the heel against the perineum, or opposite hip joint.

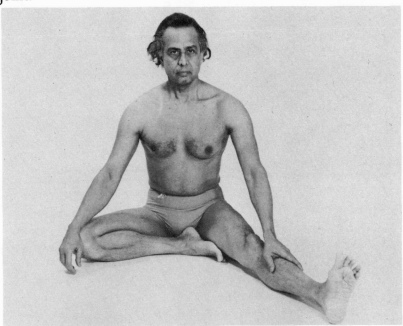

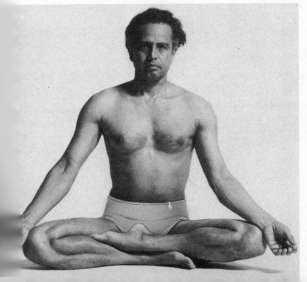

Bend the left leg and put the left foot between the right calf and thigh. Keep the arms resting loosely on the knees. The back should be kept straight, with the head, neck, and spine in a line. You can start with the right leg instead of the left if this proves more comfortable.

LOTUS POSTURE   Padmasana

The Lotus Posture is recommended as the best posture for meditation. Its benefits are those of the Easy Posture, only more pronounced.

Sit with both legs stretched. Place the right foot on the left thigh, the heel touching the root of the left thigh with the sole upturned.

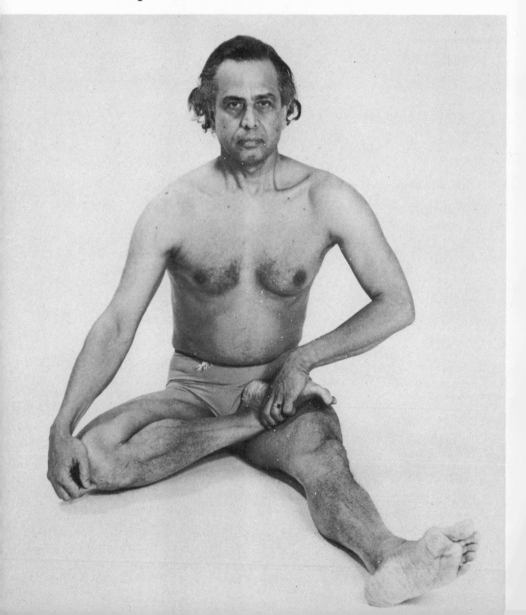

Fold the other leg and, holding the left foot with both hands, bring it over the right leg and thigh so that the heel is close to the root of the thigh. Adjust both heels so that they almost meet in front of the pelvic bones. Rest the back of your hands on the knees loosely. Or, you can put the hands together, placing the back of the left hand on the heels and the back of the right on the palm of the left.

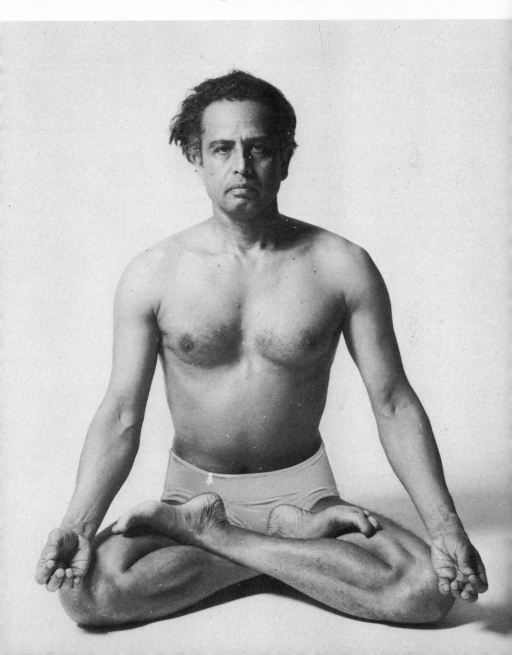

BOUND LOTUS POSE   Baddhapadmasana

This is an excellent exercise for chest and posture.

After assuming the Lotus Posture, put your hands behind your back and hold the right toe with the left hand and the left toe with the right hand.

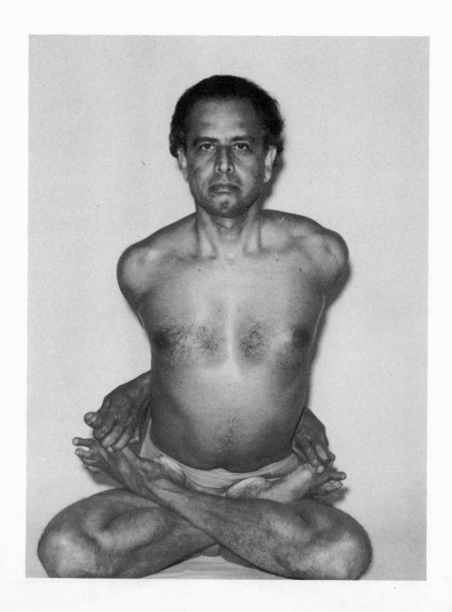

ABDOMINAL-DIAPHRAGMIC BREATHING
Pranayama I

This exercises the abdominal and diaphragmic muscles, and stimulates the organs inside the abdomen. It is especially good for women for health in their menstrual period. Hospitals today recommend some variety of it for helping natural childbirth. It is also relaxing.

Lie on your back, with the knees bent to keep the abdomen relaxed. Rest your arms on the floors or place one hand on the abdomen. Hold the body still and relaxed, with attention directed to the abdominal movement. First breathe out completely through the mouth; afterward always breathe in and out through the nose.

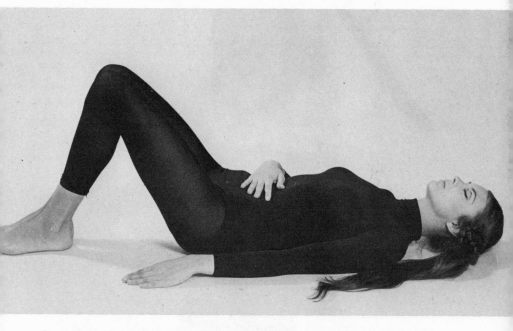

After first breathing out as indicated, breathe in slowly through the nose, pushing the abdomen out gradually without moving the chest. Breathe out immediately through the nose, slowly drawing the abdomen in as much as you can while breathing out. Suspend breath 5 to 10 seconds. Repeat the exercise 10 to 15 times.

RIBCAGE BREATHING   Pranayama II

Apart from increasing lung power, this exercise develops the intercostal muscles. It is useful for speakers and singers who need a large volume of inhaled air for sustained articulation.

Hold the ribs with both hands so that you are aware of the area involved. Breathe out completely through the mouth, then breathe in through the nose, expanding the ribs as much as possible. Keep the abdomen flat or indrawn and avoid breathing with the upper chest. After breathing in, hold the breath in for 5 to 10 seconds. As you breathe out, feel the ribs collapsing while you squeeze out the air with the action of the rib muscles. Without stopping, breathe in again and repeat the exercise 10 times.

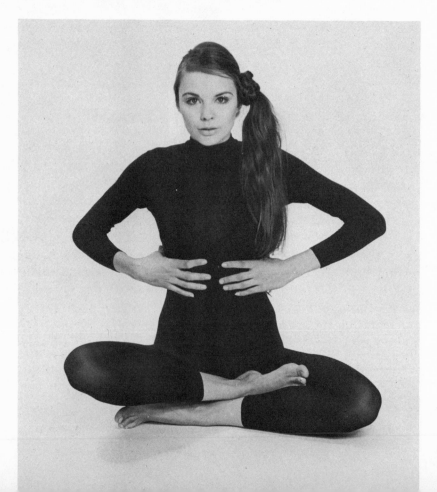

COLLARBONE BREATHING   Pranayama III

This breathing exercise helps to build broad and square shoulders. The upper areas of the lungs generally remain stagnant and become easily infected. Collarbone breathing activates these areas.

Sit in the Easy Posture or the Lotus Posture. Breathe out first through the mouth. Keep the arms loose and relaxed. Keep the abdomen flat or slightly indrawn and imagine that the ribcage is held tight by a metal vise. As you breathe in through the nose, concentrate your attention on the collarbone and shoulder area and feel that you are filling the upper areas of the lungs and that the hollow place above the collarbones is expanding. Take a couple of sniffs at the end, working the muscles in and around the neck area. Hold the air for 7 seconds. Repeat 5 to 10 times. If you feel a little dizzy at the beginning, pause and rest before resuming this exercise. If dizziness persists when you practice this exercise, do not continue it without the assistance of a practiced teacher.

COMPLETE BREATHING A   Pranayama IV

Regular practice and complete breathing will deepen the breath, eliminate faulty and rapid breathing, and have beneficial effects on the heart, the nerves, the voice, and the general appearance. It will also help you to catch your breath quickly after any strenuous effort.

Sit in the Easy Posture or the Lotus Posture, with the hands resting limp on the knees, keeping the shoulders loose and free. Empty the lungs first through the mouth. Then breathe slowly through the nose, pushing the abdomen out gently, and continue to breathe with the chest, while drawing the abdomen in in a fluid and uninterrupted movement. Breathe in as deep as you can till you feel that you are full to the brim with air. Hold the breath in for 10 to 15 seconds, and breathe out as slowly as you can. Pause after exhalation (2 to 3 seconds) and repeat 10 times. After more practice, increase the stopping time after exhalation to 5 or 6 seconds.

COMPLETE BREATHING B　　Pranayama V

Sit in the Easy Posture or the Lotus Posture. Hold the abdomen flat and start breathing until you inflate the chest fully and only then (at the end of the breathing) relax the abdomen and let it out. The rest of this exercise is the same as Complete Breathing A regarding the count and stoppage.

ABSOLUTE SUSPENSION　　Pranayama VI

This breathing has an excellent effect on the lungs, the heart, the nerve centers, the glands, and the organs in the thoracic-abdominal regions.

Lie supine with hands against the thighs, or sit in the Easy Posture with hands pressed against the knees. Empty the lungs completely through the mouth, suspend the breath, and pull in the abdomen as hard as you can so that you have a hollow below the ribs. Press the belly against the lower back and at the same time contract the anal sphincters. Hold contractions as long as you can without undue strain, then relax the abdomen and take a slow deep breath through the nose. Repeat 3 to 5 times.

BELLOWS BREATHING　　Kapalabhati

This breathing exercise is wonderful for maintaining a healthy condition of the sinuses. It is unparalleled as an exercise for oxygenation. Its effect on nerve, circulatory, and digestive systems is considerable. It has an important place in the daily physical culture program.

Sit in the Easy Posture or the Lotus Posture. Keeping the chest under control, breathe out actively with a quick, sudden and forceful contraction of the abdominal muscles. After each forceful expulsion of air with the pumplike action of a bellows, the abdomen is relaxed and inhalation takes place passively, without effort. Continue the rapid breathing as long as you can without pausing between breaths. In the beginning, practice one or two such rounds of about 30 exhalations.

SPECIAL CHEST BREATHING   Ujjayai

Ujjayai *is a powerful exercise for the chest.*

Sit in the Easy Posture or the Lotus Posture. Expel all breath through the mouth. Hold the abdomen under control and breathe in through the nose by partially closing the glottis but keeping the nostrils open and relaxed (the partial closure of the glottis will cause a sobbing sound during inhalation). Breathe in smoothly and continuously with the chest as long as you easily can, keeping the abdomen flat. After a full inhalation, close both nostrils with your fingers and hold the breath in as long as you easily can; then, breathe out through the left nostril, keeping the glottis partially closed. Repeat the exercise and exhale through the right nostril. Practice the exercise 3 times and gradually increase to 7.

ALTERNATE NOSTRIL BREATHING
Pranayama with Kumbhaka

This exercise calms the nerves and helps meditation.

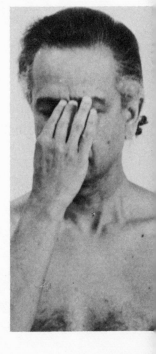

Sit in the Easy Posture or Lotus Posture, putting the back of the left hand on the left knee. Close the right nostril with the right thumb, placing the index and middle fingers on the bridge of the nose and keeping the ring and little fingers free of contact. Breathe in through the left nostril to the slow count of 4, close the left nostril also by using the little and ring fingers. Hold the breath for 8 counts, or if you can for 12 or 16 counts, then open the right nostril and breathe out to the count of 6 or 8. Breathe in again through the right nostril to the count of 4, close both nostrils and hold the breath for 8, 12, or 16 counts as before. Breathe out through the left nostril for 6 or 8 counts as before. This makes one round. Do 3 such rounds in the beginning, and increase the number of rounds gradually. Sit quiet and still, and keep your mind on the breath.

FLOOR POSTURES

COBRA POSTURE   Bhujangasana

This is a simple but excellent exercise for the spine and the abdomen. It relieves tension and expands the chest.

Lie prone on the floor in a relaxed manner with arms along your sides, the forehead or chin touching the floor and the soles turned upward.

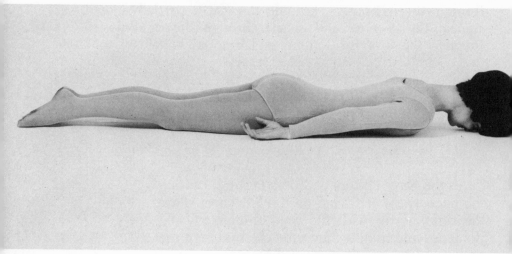

Raise your head, bending the neck back as far as possible while throwing out the chin. With the head swung back lift your chest by contracting the deep muscles of your back.

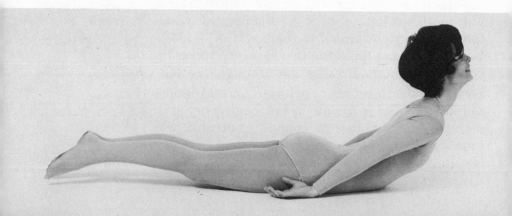

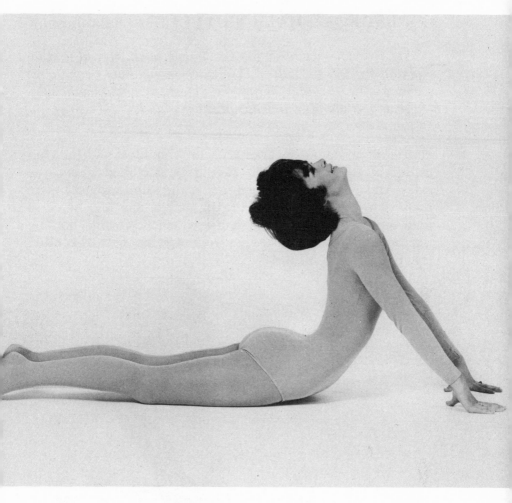

Put the palms of your hands on the floor in front of the
shoulders, keeping the elbows at your sides. Work with the
muscles of the back and the hands and curve back, gradually
lifting the elbows and bending the lumbar area so that you
feel the pressure in the sacrum. Bend the spine step by step,
feeling the pressure travelling down the spinal column gradually. Keep the hips on the floor. Hold the posture for a
few seconds and then lower the trunk step by step, reversing
the previous order. Breathing is normal in the beginning.
Later take a breath as you start, hold it during exercise,
and breathe out at the end. Practice 3 to 5 times.

LOCUST POSE, HALF AND FULL   Salabhasana

This is a fine exercise for the lower back, the hips, the abdomen, and the pelvis. It relieves many lower back pains and gastric troubles, improves digestion, and beneficially affects the bladder and the prostate gland.

Half: Lie prone on the floor with the shoulders and the chin or forehead resting on it, the arms stretched along the sides. Make fists and put them under the thighs or just beside them. After taking a deep breath, stiffen one leg, lift it as high as you can, and hold it a few seconds while holding the breath. Lower it slowly. Do the same with the other leg. Repeat each 3 times.

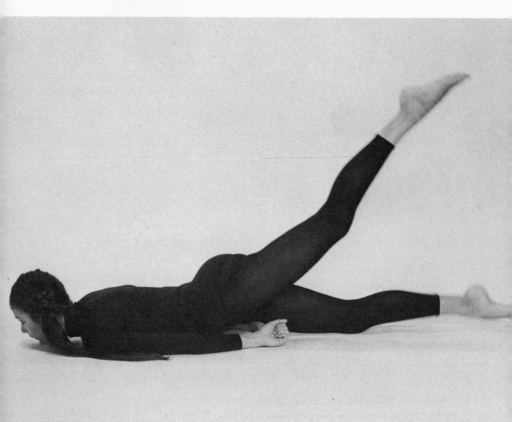

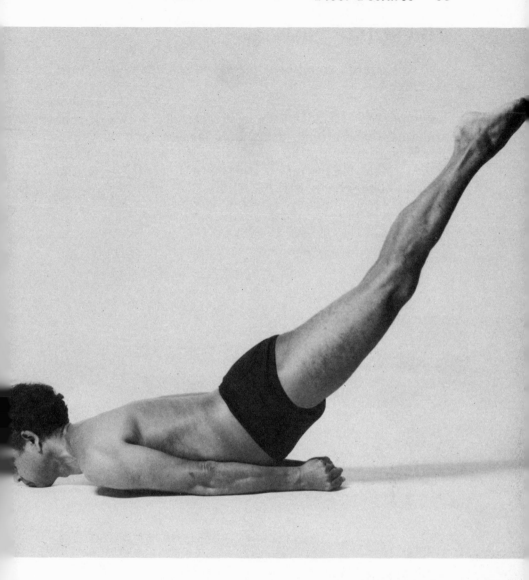

Full: Lie prone as before. Take a deep breath, stiffen the body and supporting yourself on the chest and the hands lift the legs as high as you can, lifting also the pelvic bones from the floor. Hold the position as long as you hold your breath, then lower the body, relax, and exhale. This posture is done with a sudden but smooth movement. Repeat 3 times.

THE SWING Dolasana

This exercise strengthens the back, shoulders, and hips.

Lie prone on the floor with arms extended forward. Inhale and raise head, trunk, arms, and legs as high as you can slowly and maintain the position for a few seconds. Exhale, return to the first position and relax. Repeat 3 to 5 times.

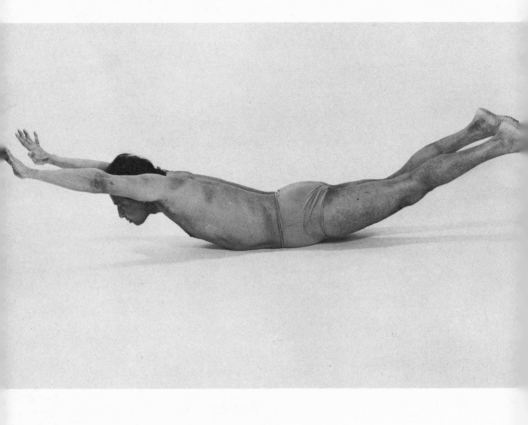

THE BOW, HALF AND FULL   Dhanurasana

The Bow stretches the abdominal section and the muscles that flex the hip-joints. It brings elasticity back to the stiff spine.

Half: Lie prone on the floor with the arms stretched over-head and chin resting on the floor. Raise arms, legs, and head as in the Swing Posture. Bend the right knee, grasp the ankle with the right hand, and pull up the knee from the floor as high as you can. Change to the other side. Alternate 3 or 4 times.

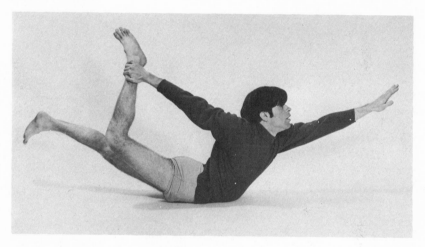

Full: Lie prone on the floor as be-fore, bend legs at the knees, grasp both ankles, and raise the trunk as well as the knees from the floor as high as you can. The whole body should rest mostly on the abdomen and curve upwards both ways like a bow. Hold the pose for about 5 seconds, then lower the chest and the knees. Finally let go the hands and put them along the sides. Breathe in before you assume the pose, after which breathing should flow nor-mally. Do it 3 to 4 times.

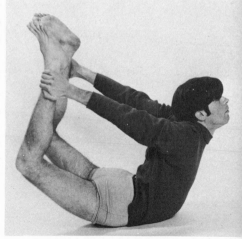

BACK STRETCHING POSE   Pashchimatanasana

This exercise is beneficial for the back muscles and the abdomen apart from its effect on the spine, especially the lumbo-sacral area. It also fully stretches and relaxes the hamstring muscles back of the knees. It tones up the nerves in the pelvic and lumbo-sacral area by bringing a greater blood supply to them. Held for a long time it has great spiritual significance.

Lie on your back with the arms stretched on the floor over your head. Keep the legs close together.

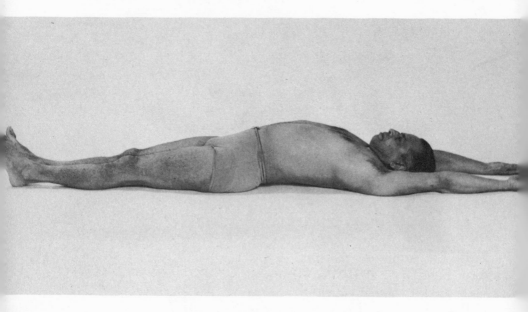

Take a deep breath, stiffen the body and, holding your breath, sit up without lifting the legs. Try to get up while keeping the head between the arms.

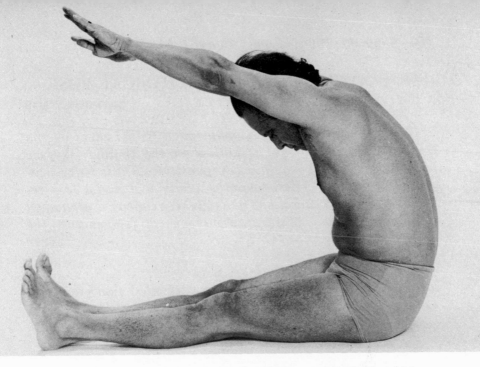

Breathe out as you bend forward and down. Hold the ankles with both hands, keep the legs straight and bring the face down slowly to the knees, bending the lumbo-sacral, lower back area, and lower the elbows to the floor. Hold a few seconds.

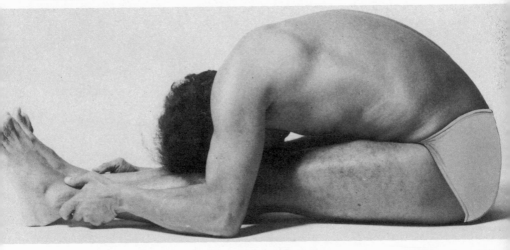

An advanced way of doing the bending is to grab the big toes with the fingers. Don't get discouraged if at first you can't bend or get up properly. Try to maintain a steady but slow pull while bending. Pull forward from the hips like folding a hinge. Repeat 3 to 4 times.

SHOULDERSTAND, OR PANPHYSICAL POSE
Sarvangasana

This exercise is highly recommended for its effect on the whole body through its action on the thyroid, the sex glands, and the abdominal organs. Many discomforts involving throat, chest, and the abdominal organs are relieved by this exercise. The yogis recommend a prolonged holding of this posture as a means of rejuvenating the body.

Lie on the floor relaxed, with arms stretched along the sides and palms on the floor.

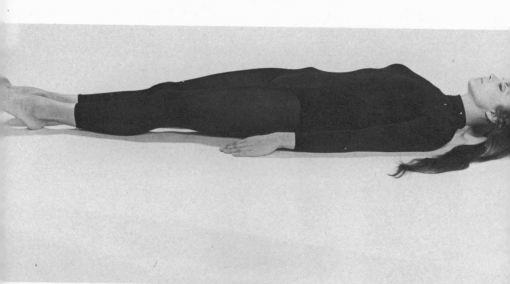

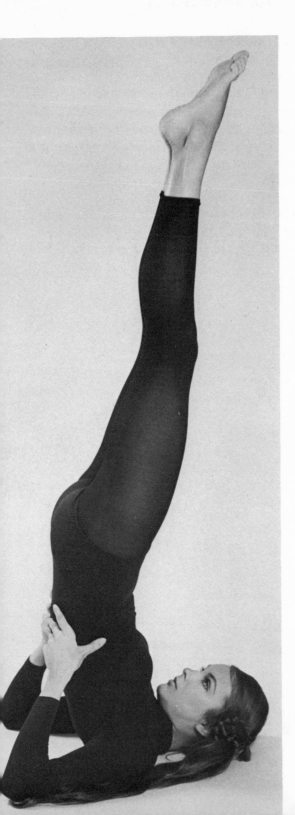

Raise the legs slowly through the hip joint and, pressing with your hands, raise the whole body with the legs thrown up while supporting the upper back with your hands. Press the chin against the Adam's apple or chest, and make the body rest on the shoulders. Hold the position for a few seconds in the beginning and then continue gradually for a longer period up to 2 or 3 minutes.

PLOW POSE   Halasana

The Plow Pose is regarded as a rejuvenating exercise, keeping the spine and the spinal nerves wonderfully healthy. It also strengthens the abdominal muscles and has a desirable effect on the thyroid and the abdominal organs. It is very relaxing, especially when the knees are bent on two sides of the head.

Lie on back with arms stretched along the sides and palms down. Raise legs slowly from the hip joint and then bring them over your head lifting the hip and the trunk.

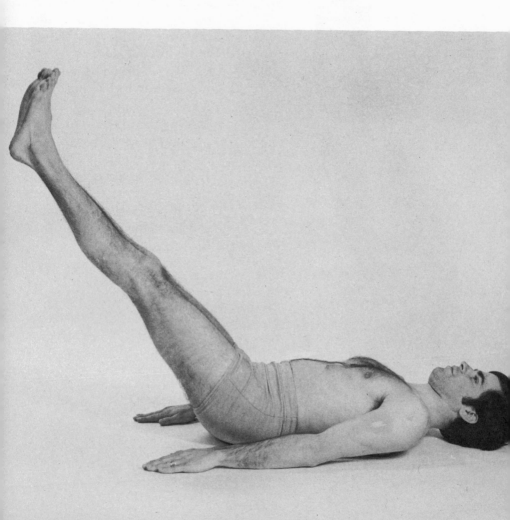

Gradually lower the toes to the floor, keeping the legs to-gether. After holding this for a while push the toes further and further away from the head until pressure is felt in the dorsal area of the spine.

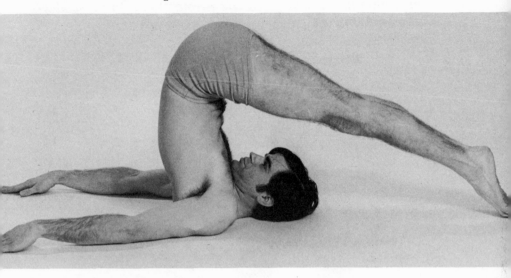

Bend the knees and bring them close to your ears. Hold the posture for a few seconds to start with and then roll forward slowly till you bring your body back to the starting position. Keep the legs straight when entering and coming out of the exercise, and move without jerks or bouncing.

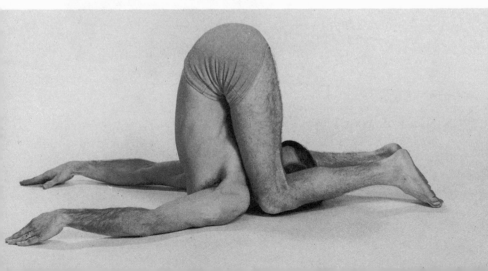

CAMEL POSE   Ushtrasana

With the practice of this exercise the abdominal and the the thigh muscles are fully stretched, while the bowels, the abdominal viscera, and the pelvic organs are considerably stimulated.

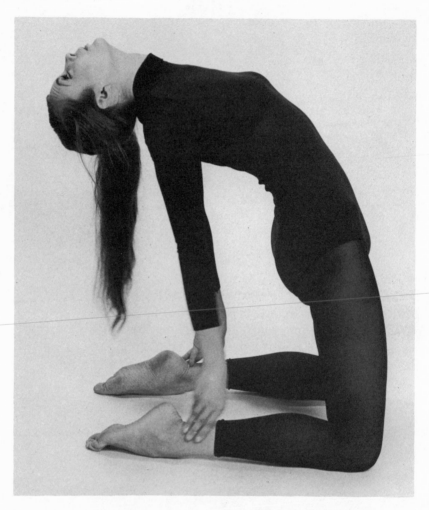

Stand on your knees, bend back keeping the thighs straight, and hold the ankles with both hands. Lower head as much as you can. Stay for a few seconds. Return to original position. Repeat 2 or 3 times. Breathing should be normal.

SUPINE PELVIC POSE   Supta Vajrasana

Kneel on the floor with legs apart and gradually lower your seat to the floor between the feet. Lie back with the help of your elbows.

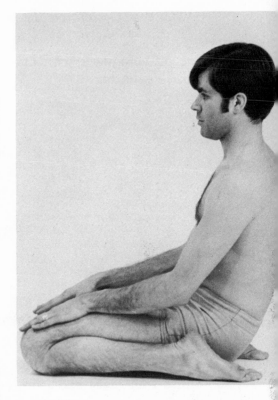

Put your palms on the thighs and arch your back fully. Breathing should be normal.

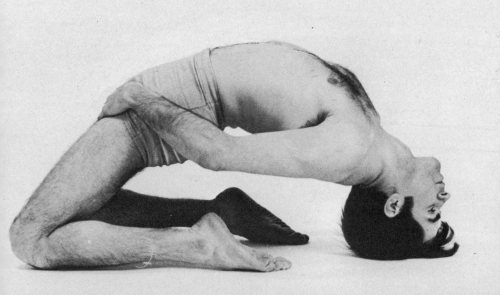

THE WHEEL   Chakrasana

The Wheel exercises the shoulders, chest, abdomen, lower back, and the face.

Lie on your back with knees bent, and the feet apart but close to the body.

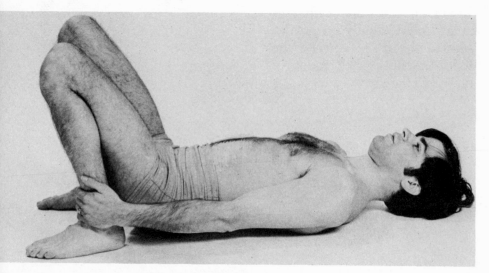

Raise your body like a bridge resting it on the feet and the head, gradually narrowing the distance between feet and head.

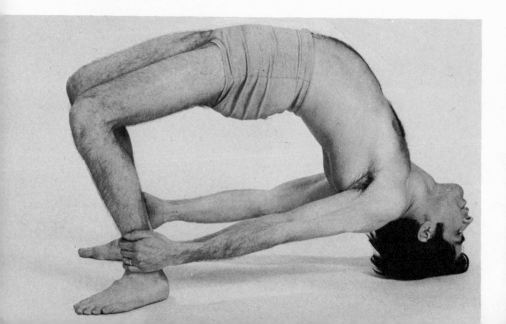

Release the grip from your ankles, bend your arms, and put the palms of the hands on the floor near the shoulders with the fingers pointing to them. Continue to arch your back, pushing up and raising yourself as high as possible from the floor.

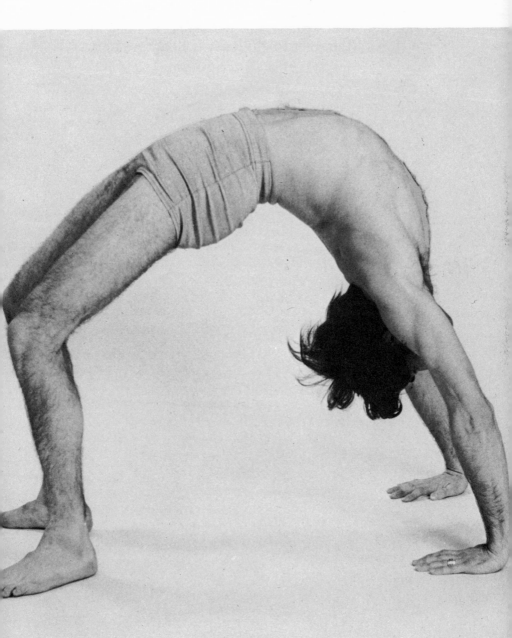

HEAD KNEE POSTURE   Janusirasana

The exercise benefits are similar to the Back Stretching Pose. It further helps in loosening the hip joints.

Sit on floor with legs stretched out. Bend the left knee and bring the heel against the perineum, keeping the sole in touch with the right thigh. Raise both arms.

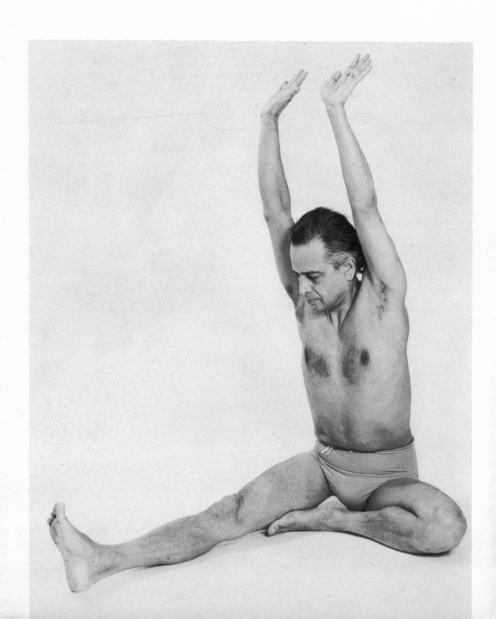

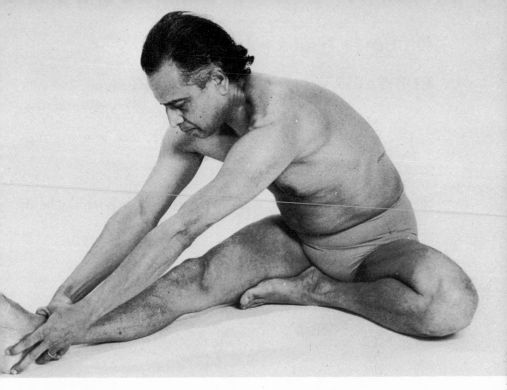

Bend body forward and downward, and hold the right ankle or foot with both hands.

Bring the face down to the knee of the right leg, and pull the elbows down to the floor. Hold this position for a few seconds and return to the seated position with both feet outstretched. Exhale as you bend down and inhale as you resume the first position. Repeat 2 times on each side.

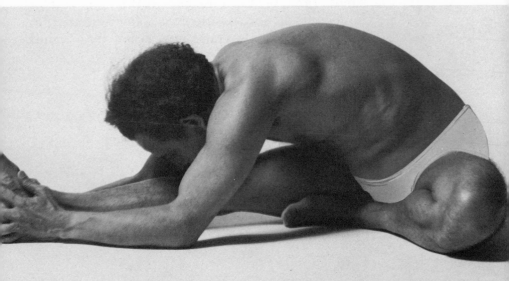

FORWARD HEAD-BEND POSTURE
Bhunamanasana

This posture is excellent for the lower back and the hip joints.

Sit with legs stretched and apart as far as possible, and raise both arms.

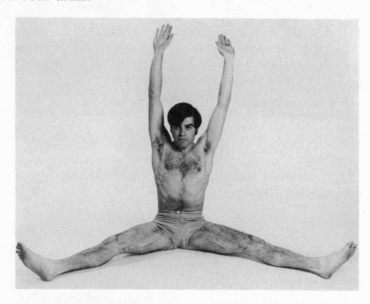

Bend down and forward, and grasp the soles of the feet with the hands, bringing the forehead to the floor without bending the legs. Hold this position for a few seconds. Repeat 2 times. Inhale as you come up, raising both hands. Exhale as you go down.

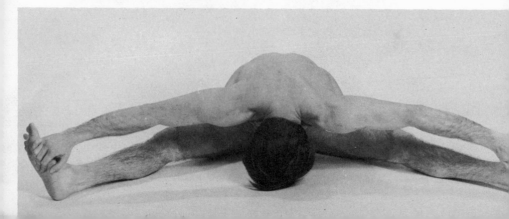

HEADSTAND   Sirshasana

The Headstand is regarded as the master posture by the yogis. It sends a circulating supply of blood to the brain, promotes the health of the whole nervous system, and preserves and heightens the efficiency of the organs of sight, smell, hearing, and taste by stimulating their different centers located in the brain. It improves the functioning of all the important endocrine glands situated above the heart, pineal, pituitary, thyroid, and parathyroid, by supplying them with an increased supply of fresh blood. It has an important and beneficial effect on the digestive system and the abdominal organs. In short, the Headstand is excellent for preserving general health and promoting organic vigor.

Kneel on the floor, put your head down, and cup your hands with fingers interlocked against the head. Don't spread the elbows too wide apart.

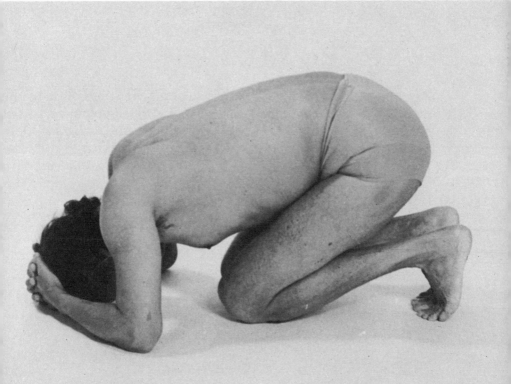

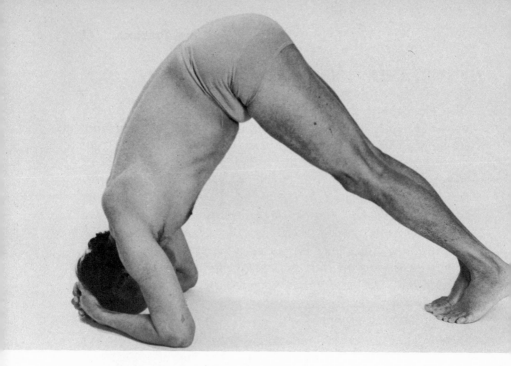

Raise your hips, and straighten your legs and back.

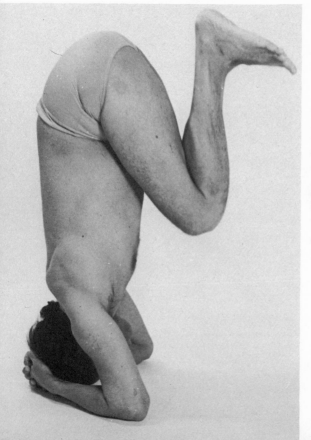

Bring the knees close to the chest, raising your feet from the ground with a little push, working with the lower back just as you would hop to ride a bicycle.

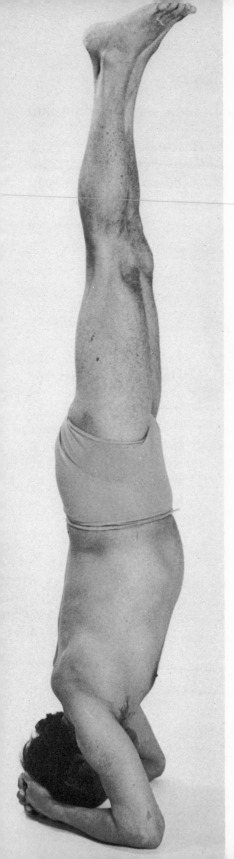

Balance yourself with legs bent and then slowly raise the legs up. Think of the lower back and the spine and keep your weight mostly on the elbows. Practice against a wall or a sofa in the beginning if you are alone, or let somebody help you. Stay in position for a few seconds to begin with. Increase gradually up to 5 minutes.

HEADSTAND WITH LOTUS POSE
Shirshasana with Padmasana

This is an advanced form of the Headstand Posture. Before you can do the Headstand with Lotus Pose you must learn to sit in the Lotus Posture easily and properly for a span of time.

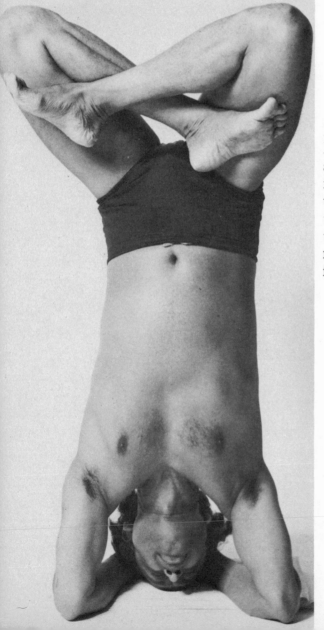

Proceed as for the Headstand. When you are comfortably and firmly in position, fold the left leg and place the foot over the right thigh, then fold the right leg and place the foot over the left thigh.

MOUNTAIN POSTURE Parvatasana

This exercise improves balance, while strengthening the lower back and the hips.

Assume the Lotus Pose. Using your hands as supports, stand on your knees. Then raise your hands and join them together over your head.

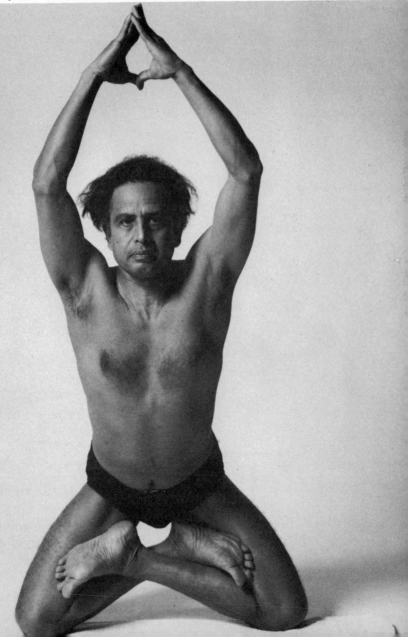

SPINAL SIDE TWISTS   Ardhamatsyendrasana

This posture bends and twists the spine on both sides, invigorating the nerve centers in the spine through muscular contraction and accelerated blood supply.

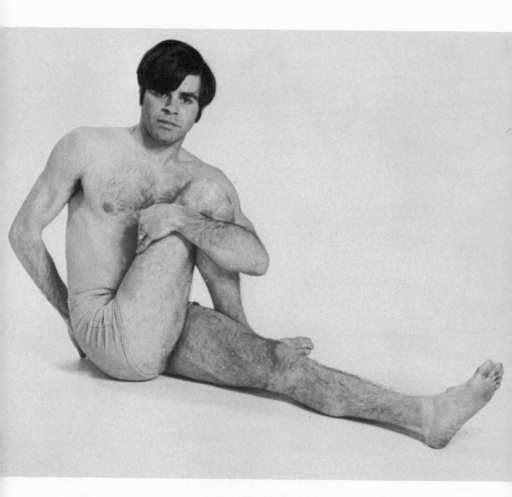

Sit with your legs stretched and bending the right leg move it over the left leg, pressing the right heel against the left thigh. Bend the left leg and place the left foot under the right hip. Place the right knee under the left arm pit, while holding the right knee with your left hand. Then swing the right arm behind the back, and twisting the back, head, and shoulders, touch or hold the right ankle with your right hand. The head should turn right as far as possible and the chin should be above the right shoulder. The chest should be straight. Hold the posture for a few seconds. Then do the reverse. Do it 2 or 3 times on each side. Breathing should remain normal.

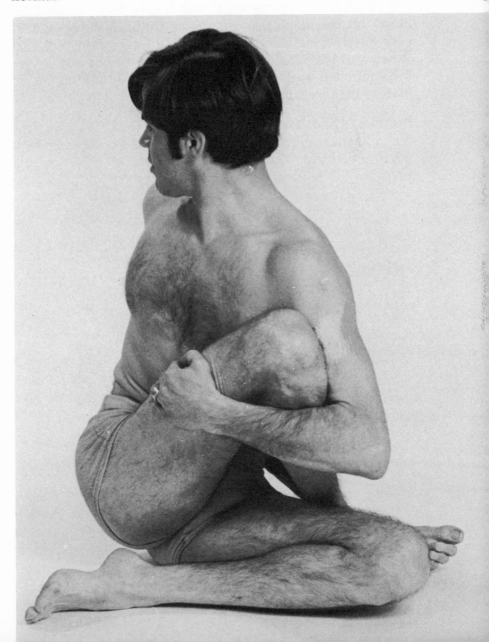

STOMACH LIFT   Uddiyana

The Uddiyana *and* Nauli *Postures are best done in the morning on an empty stomach.*

Sit in any of the postures for meditation, the Easy or the Lotus (the Stomach Lift can also be practiced while standing). Place the hands on the knees. Empty the lungs with full exhalation and, pressing your hands firmly against the knees, lift the diaphragm up aiming to touch the spine with your navel. Bend your head, bringing the chin to the chest. When you find you cannot hold the breath out any longer, relax the neck and shoulders, lower the ribs, and take a full breath. Do this 3 to 5 times.

Further, while holding the breath out, you can also relax and lift your abdomen and ribs repeatedly, flapping as in mock breathing. This is a superior form of *Uddiyana* and prepares the student for the *Nauli* posture.

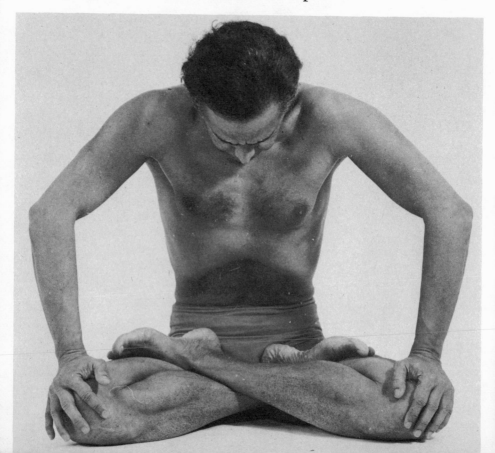

ISOLATION OF ABDOMINAL RECTI   Nauli

Uddiyana and Nauli are regarded as excellent exercises for sex control and for absorption of the secretions of the gonads into the bloodstream to help in the reconstruction of the body and continuation of youthfulness.

Stand with your feet nearly a foot apart and, bending forward slightly from the waist, place your hands on the thighs near the groin or the knees. (This can also be done sitting or kneeling, but it is best done standing.) Bend the knees slightly. Exhale fully, draw the abdomen in and up. Pressing your hands on the thighs or knees, isolate and push forward the rectus muscles. The two sides of the abdomen will remain soft and hollow while the middle portion should be hard and raised. Practice of the Stomach Lift with a flapping motion will help to bring about this condition.

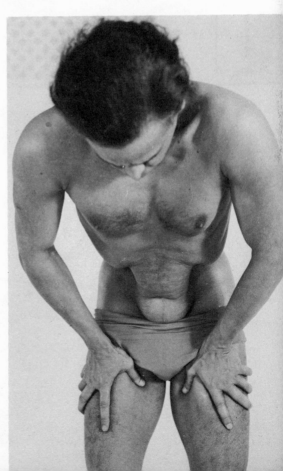

After you have practiced the central *Nauli*, try the left and right *Naulis* by manipulating the muscles separately. In doing these you must lean to one side, i.e., while isolating the right rectus lean toward the right and while isolating the left rectus lean to the left. Next roll the muscles from one side to the other with a swaying motion of the body.

HIP STAND   Nitambasana

This exercise strengthens the hip muscles, and improves their flexibility.

Sit with your legs together and stretched before you on the floor. As you lean back, lift both legs and touch the toes with outstretched arms.

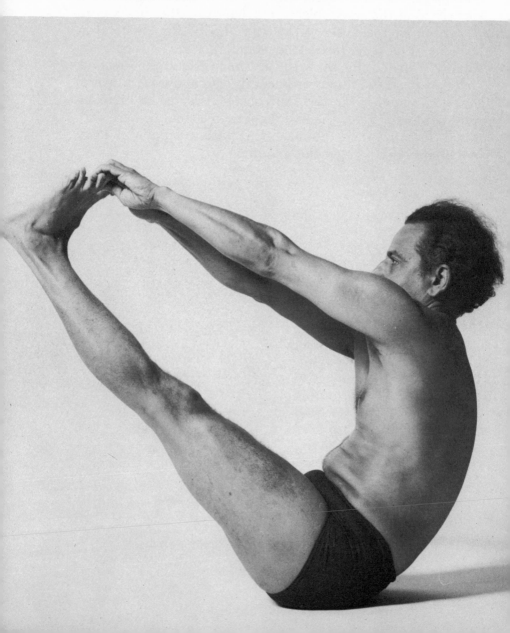

FISH POSTURE   Matsyasana

This is a complementary exercise to the Panphysical Pose.

Assume the Lotus Posture. Lie on your back while keeping the knees down. With the aid of your elbows, arch your back and throw the head backward, making a bridge with your seat and head. Grasp the toes with your forefingers.

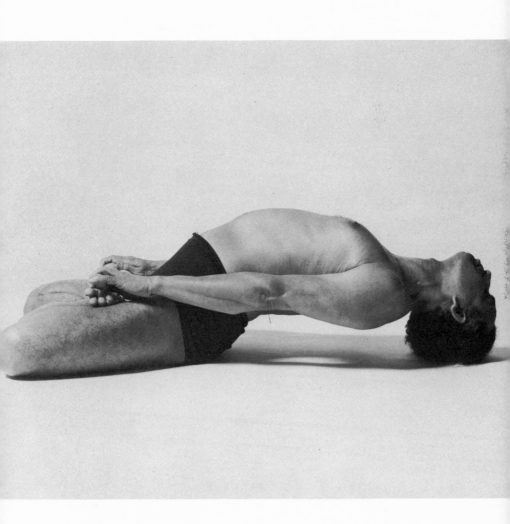

LATERAL LIFT   Parshvasana

This exercise strengthens the lower back and hip muscles.

Lie on your side, as in the Lateral Spine Posture, and lift both legs as high as you can from the floor, keeping your heels together.

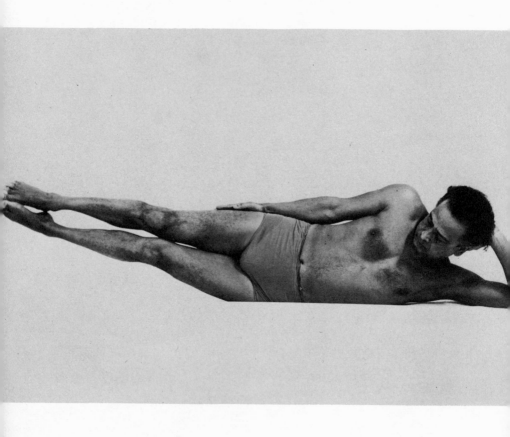

LATERAL SPINE POSTURE
Parsva Merudandasana

This exercise stretches and strengthens the lateral muscles of the back and abdomen, and enhances flexibility of the trunk.

Lie on your right side, with the trunk, hip, and legs in a straight line. Place the left arm on the left side, with the hand on the thigh. Support the head with the right hand, with the right elbow resting on the floor. Slowly raise your head and trunk laterally as much as you can without lifting your legs. Do the same exercise on the alternate side. Breathing should remain normal throughout.

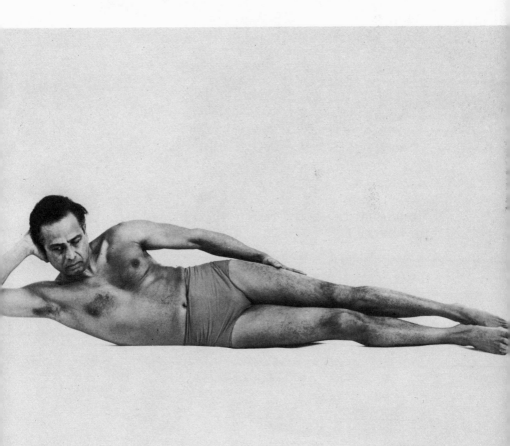

THE PEACOCK   Mayurasana

The Peacock Pose tones the digestive system and protects against the drooping of the abdominal organs. It also invigorates the nervous system.

Kneel with palms on the floor, with the fingers pointed back toward the body, and with the elbows under the ribs and abdomen.

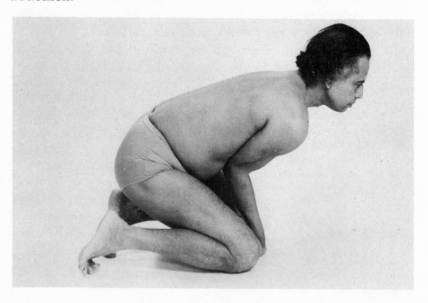

Stretch out the body, resting the ribs and the abdomen on the elbows.

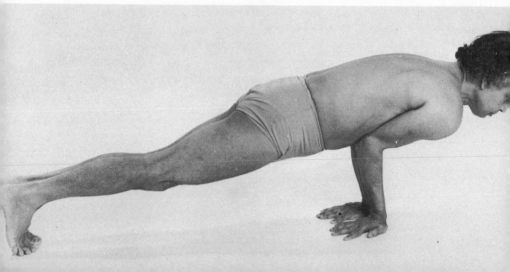

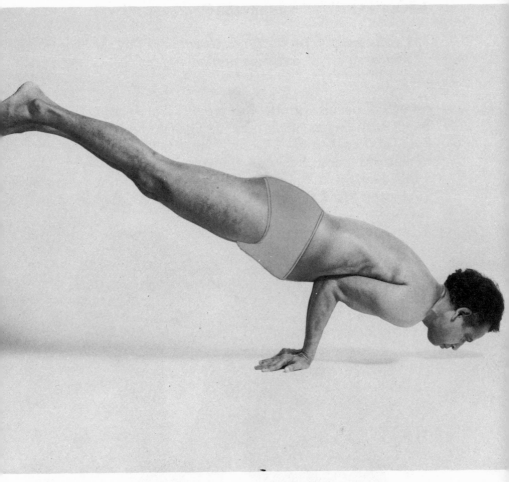

Lean forward and raise the feet from the floor, lifting them
up gradually.

LION POSE   Simhasana

This is an exercise for chest, throat, and face. It helps prevent crow's-feet wrinkles around the corners of the eyes.

Sit on your heels with the feet crossed. Put your hands on the knees with fingers open, pressing against the knees. Draw in your abdomen and, lowering your head, press the chin against the chest. Stick out your tongue as much as possible while looking at the point between the eyebrows, crossing your eyes. Hold this position a few seconds. Repeat several times.

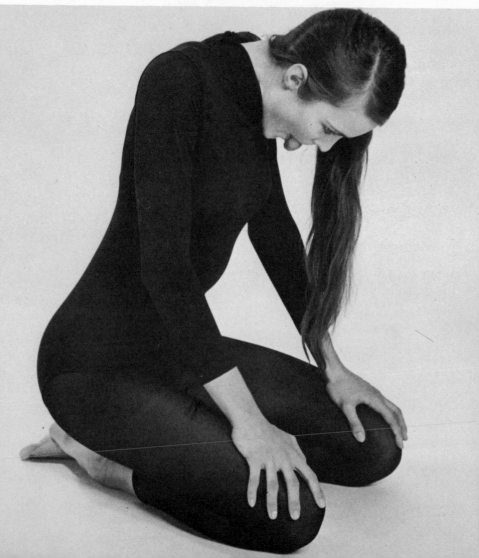

THE SYMBOL OF YOGA   Yoga Mudra

This is an excellent pelvic exercise. It builds a powerful abdominal wall, helping to keep the organs in their proper place. It also tones the nervous system in general and the lumbo-sacral nerves in particular.

Sit in the Lotus Posture. Fold your hands behind, holding them together. Bend forward and, pressing the heels against the abdomen, touch the floor with the forehead. Don't jerk but bend slowly, and don't get discouraged if you cannot touch the floor with your head in the beginning. Do as much bending as you can without bouncing or jerky movements. Hold a few seconds.

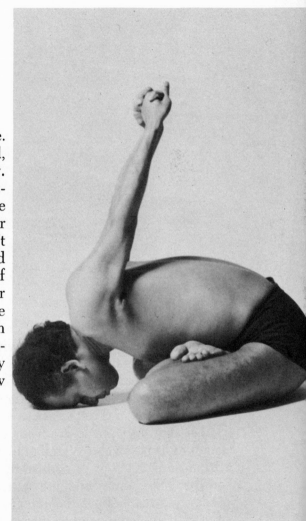

THE DEAD POSE   Savasana

*The Dead Pose is for relaxation at the end of the exercise.
It can be practiced at other times, also, with great benefit.
The practice of this pose has a very relaxing and calming
effect on the nerves.*

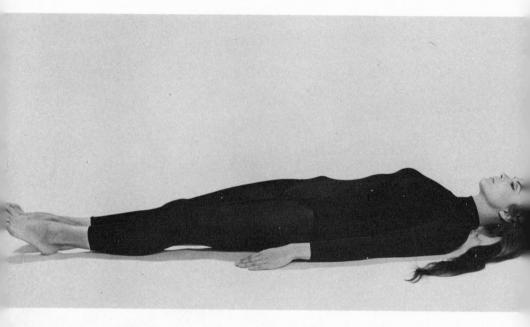

On a light mattress or a thick carpet spread on a hard and
even surface, lie on your back with the arms resting on the
floor with the palms up. Close your eyes. Consciously relax
the different parts of the body starting from the feet. Feel
that you have let the body go completely and that it lies limp
and motionless and detached, as it were, from the mind.

Feel that you are apart from the body and that you are
watching it passively. Watch your breath as it goes in and out
without any attempt to control it.

After some time, imagine you are inhaling and exhaling
a silvery stream. Feel the stream going through every part
of your body from head to toes as you inhale. As you breathe
in, imagine you are gaining health and strength, poise and
calmness; as you exhale, imagine you are throwing out all
tired feelings, all restlessness, all fears and anxieties. Repeat
a few times. Practice 10 minutes or so.

3

HEALTH
FOOD
MEDITATION
CONCLUSION

Save the self by the self, never depress the self. Self is one's best friend as well as the worst enemy.

The Gita

HEALTH,

YOUTHFULNESS,

AND APPEARANCE

Health needs attention to a host of factors; exercise, food, rest including fasting, positive thoughts, and emotional balance.

In the long run, health which is not mental health turns out to be no health at all. In affluent communities—which do not lack food and vitamins, sport and activity, leisure and entertainment—the diseases are predominantly of emotional origin. Yogis hold that heart disease and arthritis, which are the common killers and cripplers today, are mostly emotionally induced.

Emotional balance cannot be attained without cultivation of positive thoughts and pursuit of right values. As our body needs vitamins and minerals to be strong and healthy, so also does our mind need positive thoughts and values to keep it healthy and dynamic.

Pursuit of materialistic values as the ultimate is the disease of worldliness against which spiritual teachers warn us. What are spiritual values and what is spirituality? Spiritual values are Truth, Love, Freedom; spirituality is pursuit of them. Spirituality is striving for the manifestation of the divine essence of man. Man has his specific perfection, as plants and animals have their specific excellences; it is the manifestation of the real man in us, our abiding character. We come to dead ends by chasing materialistic goals; if we do not see their limitations, if we fail to pursue the true end of life for which other goals are means and fail to realize that our fulfilment lies in the transcendence of our limited and finite individualistic life, we can never be free from fear, anxiety, insecurity, tension, and a sense of incompleteness.

It is the pursuit of idealism which keeps the mind young. Old age is stiffness of body and mind. To retain youthfulness of body, we have to pay attention not only to the physical factors but to mental attitudes as well. A youthful and dynamic mind is characterized by growth, hope, and aspiration for higher spiritual goals. Calm emotions, hope and dynamism in life keep persons healthy and vigorous. The kind of thoughts we think mark and mold our face. Emotions and atttitudes manifest themselves in our body as years go by. In later years conditions of the psyche, its hope and despair, its serenity and tension, all reveal themselves in health or disease, in comeliness or ugliness. Good thoughts and warm feelings, love and peacefulness, bring new qualities to our looks. For men of taste, a face which does not reveal goodness and warmth, simplicity and purity, has no attraction.

Meditation on the truth of self is the best means of achieving calmness of mind. We need a proper outlook in life, an outlook based on the deeper truth of existence.

FOOD

Attention to food and eating habits is of prime importance for health, long life, youthful appearance, and also for therapeutic reasons. This is especially so in opulent communities where food is plentiful in variety and richness, where temptations are too many and easily indulged in, and where natural taste has been corrupted by artificial processing of food.

The question of food is complex, depending upon the individual's climate and background, but some general principles derived from reason and long experience can be laid down.

In communities where food is abundant the first principle

is that of moderation. People usually overeat. Overeating, apart from leading to overweight and consequent bad effects, deposits a lot of surplus waste material in the body and the body gets sick in the effort to expel the toxic substances.

One should cut down on his intake of food after the age of 35. We have food for growth, for fuel purposes, and for repairing of the wear and tear of the tissues of the body. We cease to grow after the age of 30 or so, and our physical activity also declines with age. However, the old eating habits not only persist but change for the worse. People eat and drink more, especially the wrong foods and drinks.

The acids and waste products—the metabolic debris—in the blood and tissue fluids are expelled less easily from the body of a grownup person. The aging process is hastened in the case of individuals who overeat.

Food should be cut down when we reach middle age. There should be good intervals between eating. Stomach and other organs need rest.

Periodic fasting once a week or fortnight is beneficial for grown-ups. It cleanses the body and restores vitality. Take plenty of fluids, fruit juices, or lemon water with a pinch of salt while you fast. If you feel hungry at the end of the day, have a light vegetable meal—fresh boiled vegetables—in the evening. Extensive fastings and change of food habits should be undertaken under expert advice.

Food should be fresh and clean. Avoid as much as you can the processed and chemically preserved foods. Greasy and fried foods are bad for adults.

It is good to reduce, or give up altogether if possible, meat eating as one grows in years. Fresh fish is an excellent substitute for meat, especially under modern conditions.

Personal feeling and considerations of health are two reasons behind the practice of vegetarianism. In later years and especially for persons of intellectual pursuits, a vegetarian diet is helpful.

Weight should be controlled by proper natural diet, exercise, and fasting. It is injurious to take pills and to take artificial foods which claim to provide the required minimum calories for physical health and maintenance. People may lose weight by means of pills, but they often lose their minds, too, as a side effect!

One can be sure of a healthy diet if one keeps to the following kinds of food: fresh vegetables and salads, fruits, fresh fish (boiled or broiled), vegetable oils, yogurt, lemon, honey, whole wheat, and rice.

One should feel really hungry before eating. It is not good to fuss too much about calories or to be a faddist about food. Moderation in eating and keeping to fresh, simple food mentioned above are enough. Also, one should follow one's natural and uncorrupted taste for food. We often know instinctively what is good for us.

MEDITATION

Meditation is the essence of yoga. Yogic meditation is concentration of mind upon our higher self, the pure subjective principle in us which is neither the body nor the mind but the pure changeless, formless, and boundless awareness, the spirit or being on which the transient mental and physical changes are projected. This self or spirit is the transcendental principle or reality, above and beyond the processes of mind and body or nature. That is why meditation on self or spirit is sometimes called transcendental meditation.

It is not easy to gather the energies of mind into a sharp focus and throw them back on the self. Mind is restless like the wind. It requires long and steady practice, with faith, energy, and devotion to harness the powers of mind. However, even a little of this yoga of meditation is of immense help in promoting health and helping us to acquire better self-control and emotional stability by getting to know the deeper workings of mind.

We gain knowledge in two ways—perception, and inference or reasoning. But such knowledge is relative and practical in the narrow sense. There is a higher method of knowing reality—through meditation. There are different levels of meditation. As our mind gets calmer and purer, devoid more and more of dullness and distraction, it apprehends the subtler truths and facts which underlie gross appearances relative to our gross senses. Meditation develops the powers of subtle perception. In the highest meditation the mind is perfectly calm and still and reflects the clear image of the spirit as a tranquil sheet of water reflects the blue sky perfectly. Only then do we know what is the absolute truth, the reality behind all appearances, free from all distortion by sense or imagination.

Meditation should be a routine practice for those who are spiritually awakened and aspire after the higher values of life beyond those of material power and enjoyment. Meditation balances our life and gives it the right orientation. It helps us to see ourselves and others more clearly and objectively and to make better judgments in life. It is not only restful for our mind but beneficial for our health.

Some hints on meditation are given below.

It is necessary to have at the outset some physical aids and positive imaginations. Find a quiet and clean spot free from worldly associations where you can practice daily. It is good to have a special seat for the purpose and a few flowers and mild incense around.

Sit in an easy and relaxed posture holding the back, the neck, and the head in a line. The Easy Posture and the Lotus Posture are the best ones. If you cannot hold these postures easily, sit in a sofa with legs stretched out fully and resting on an ottoman or any other object on the same level as the seat. Keep the back supported but straight.

Sit quiet and still with eyes closed and hands resting, light and limp, on the knees or on your lap. Tell yourself that you are leaving the everyday world behind you and that you are retiring into another world, the inner world of the spirit, your true homeland, the realm of eternity, of immortal life, and of everlasting peace, strength, and bliss.

Suggest that your body is the temple of the spirit within and that it is strong and healthy in every part.

Send out thoughts of love, peace, and goodwill to all your near and dear ones and to the rest of humanity.

Offer a prayer to the Divine Spirit for health, strength, and understanding.

Do a few simple rhythmic breathings, *pranayamas*.

Then for a while be a detached and silent spectator of your mind and body. Assert that you are the pure and changeless spirit, the luminous witness apart from your thoughts and sensations. Observe all thoughts and sensations as events outside of you. Do not identify yourself with anything, but stand aloof as a pure witness.

You can continue in this meditation, or change into another and take any one object you like, the figure of a saint or prophet or a luminous presence to fix your mind on. Put the object in the heart, not the physical heart but the area where our deepest emotions are reflected, in the spine. Regard the object or the image as the visible manifestation of the infinite spirit, pure consciousness, and bliss. Hold your mind on the object or the light, steadily repeating Om, or any other *mantra,* inwardly and feel that your self has melted away into the boundless existence, consciousness, and bliss.

Meditate as long as you can without strain and get up after offering another prayer for understanding and peace.

It is good to keep a special hour for meditation.

CONCLUSION

I want to conclude with a final note about the excellence of hatha yoga for physical fitness in light of recent research. Medical doctors in a number of publications have drawn attention to research showing that physical fitness and vigor depend on efficiency of the cardiovascular system, which include the lungs, the heart, and the blood vessels. Physical fitness is the capacity for long sustained effort and endurance and derives from proper oxygenation of blood and the delivery of a rich supply of the blood to the tissues of the body. This goal is achieved by conditioning the lungs to process more air with less effort and the heart to pump more blood with less beats. And, contrary to general belief, popular gymnastics, live weight lifting, and calisthenics, isometric, and isotonic exercises are poor performers in this respect as compared with running, swimming, cycling, etc. The new system of aerobics is founded on the above findings.

It is also being recognized that a slower rate of breathing and heart beat while at rest are signs of better health and stamina. Those who are acquainted with yoga know that centuries ago the yogis emphasized that slow, restful, and rhythmic breathing promotes health and long life. The yogis developed specific exercises for improving lung and heart tone. Some time ago it was reported in the press that Soviet astronauts were being trained in yoga breathing to prepare them for long flights with less strain on their lungs and hearts.

However, the yoga system of health is more far-reaching in its approach to health problems than are the modern ones as I pointed out at the beginning.

A very important problem which a system of hygiene must take note of in modern society is tension, an all-pervasive feature of life today. Demand for relief from tension is nearly universal. Any region of health which does not provide means for such relief cannot be adequate. All physical exercises relieve tension to some extent, but the yoga stretchings and the yoga breathings are unique in this respect. Further, as mentioned earlier, yoga reaches deeper into the subtler aspects of health. This need for a more basic approach is being increasingly realized by modern medical practice.

The remarkable power of yoga in releasing new energy and making the body and mind dynamic has already been noted by some distinguished Americans. In 1909 William James, in a lecture delivered before the Philosophical Association of Columbia University entitled "The Energies of Men," described how a friend of his had attained miraculous results through the practice of yoga. The friend used to suffer from chronic depression, fatigue, and poor health. After six months of yoga practice, he was a changed person with plenty of surplus energy, needing much less rest, sleep, and food than before. The article was later published as a book under the title, *The Energies of Men and the Gospel of Relaxation.* More recently Congresswoman Frances Bolton attributed her remarkable vitality at the age of 75 to the regular practice of yoga for over half a century.

I have seen many persons who started initially with simple yoga exercises later become interested in the subtler aspects of philosophy and attitude as their awareness improved with the practice of yoga. There are thousands in America today to testify to the marvellous results they have derived from yoga; how it has improved their physical and mental well-being and given a new meaning and direction to their life.

Yoga's wide scope and the test of ages makes it the most suitable form of health culture for the civilized individual.

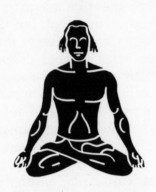

This self cannot be attained by the weak.
Upanishad